Essential Oils 101

A Beginner's Guide to Health Basics with Essential Oils

Carrie Donegan & Elena Yordán

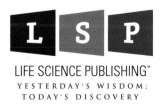

LIFE SCIENCE PUBLISHING™
YESTERDAY'S WISDOM;
TODAY'S DISCOVERY

Second Edition

Published and offered for sale by Life Science Publishing
Phone: 800-336-6308 • www.lifesciencepublishers.com

ISBN: 978-0-9835183-58

Second Edition 2013

Distributed by Diamond Circle, LLC
www.yl90plan.com

IMPORTANT

The information in this book reflects the authors' experiences and opinions and is not intended to replace medical advice.

These statements have not been evaluated by the Food and Drug Administration. These products are not intended to diagnose, treat, cure or prevent any disease.

This book has been designed to provide information to help educate the reader in regard to the subject matter covered. It is sold with the understanding that the publisher and the authors are not liable for the misconception or misuse of the information provided. It is not provided in order to diagnose, prescribe, or treat any disease, illness, or injured condition of the body. The authors and publisher shall have neither liability nor responsibility to any person or entity with respect to any loss, damage, or injury caused or alleged to be caused directly or indirectly by the information contained in this book. The information presented herein, is in now way intended as a substitute for medical counseling. Anyone suffering from any disease, illness, or injury should consult a qualified healthcare professional.

Design: Paul Springer / Bailey-Montague Graphic Design

Let not your heart be disturbed.
Do not fear that sickness, nor any other
sickness or anguish. Am I not here, who
am your Mother? Are you not under my
protection? Am I not your health?
Are you not happily within my fold?
What else do you wish? Do not grieve
nor be disturbed by anything."

—OUR LADY OF GUADALUPE TO JUAN DIEGO—

Our Mission

Most books on essential oils are written by doctors, scientists, nurses, healers, or religious who have studied plants and their medicinal uses through the eye of a microscope or the eyes of their patients. Our humble testimony here is just that—a body of experience compiled for more than a decade and from the combined experiences of more than 1,000 people who have joined us in our quest for health answers through natural solutions.

What we bring to you here is a beginning—a place to start. For each issue we have shared a possible use of essential oils and products. Are there more combinations? Of course, an unlimited number in fact. But the question that one always asks at the beginning is, "where do you start?"

We suggest you start here. Essential Oils 101. Our simple guide will give you a 90-day plan for each problem presented. The information we have is what has worked for us in our everyday lives and in those of our friends and families as well. We hope this guide will serve you as well as it has served us.

Let's keep the conversation going. Find us at: www.YL90Plan.com

Table of Contents

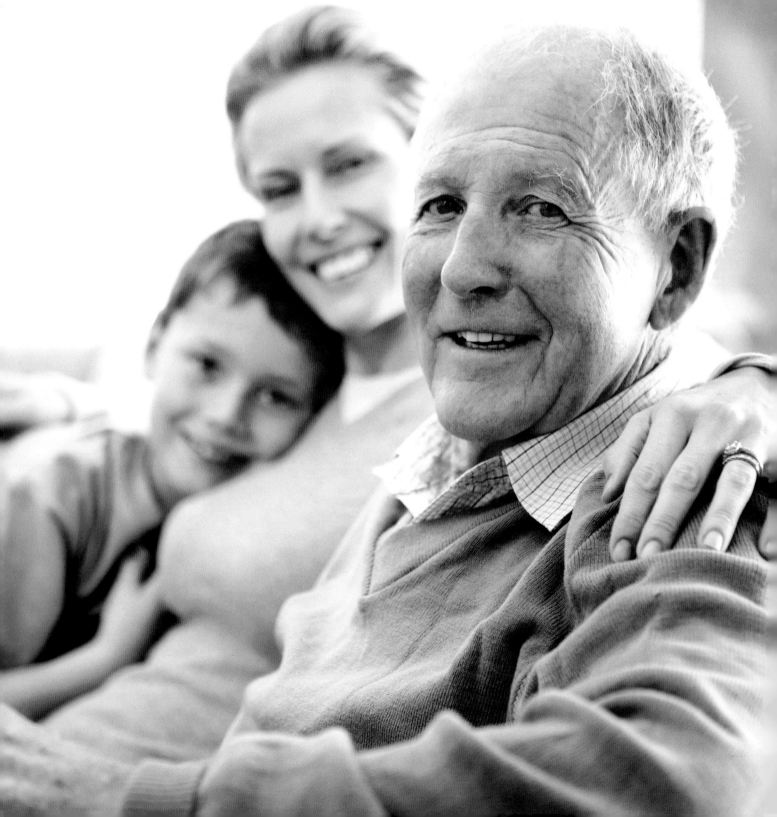

Acknowledgements

In many ways this book not only represents our experiences with essential oils and natural products it represents a gathering of people, the community we came from, and the one that grew out of our searching for information. There have been hundreds of meetings, meals, phone conversations, courses, lectures, conferences, and talks from which we have learned. There are thousands of people, across many continents, who have truly touched our lives and we value all they have done for us.

As in any experience, there are people who are indispensable. The ones who stand by you, put up with your bad days, put bandaids on your wounds, cheer you on, and pray for you. The following are those special people:

Our husbands and children: you made this book possible! You are our core; a constant source of love and inspiration. We are so grateful to you: Fred, Carrie's husband, and their two children, Rick & Ciara; José, Elena's husband, and their children Laura & Henry.

Our parents: we are both only children, raised by strong mothers, Sally Turner and Clara Ostrowski, who gave us a solid foundation, a strong faith formation, and an unwavering belief that we could do anything

that we set out to do and to never waste the gifts we have been given. Bruce Turner, Carrie's step-dad and overall good egg to both of us. To our fathers, both gone too soon, we wish you could have been here to share this book with us.

Our friends and colleagues: Ginger Andro, Natalie Amoia, Lillian Brenwasser, Glenda Coughlin, Jennifer Czuckermann, Paul Donegan, Erin Giddens, Chuck Glicksman, Christine Gehres, John Guarnieri, Claudia Hanlin, Margarete Hyer, Maia Ietta, Jan Jeremias, Karin Johnson, Barbara Kashevaroff, Francesca Lehman, Barbara Light, Mitch Mensch, Gina McConeghy, Jennifer Minicus, Maria Morocho, Mary Moscarello, Ellis Orsay, Nick Orsay, Karen Overgaard RN,

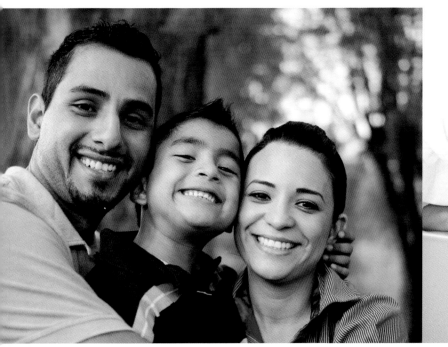
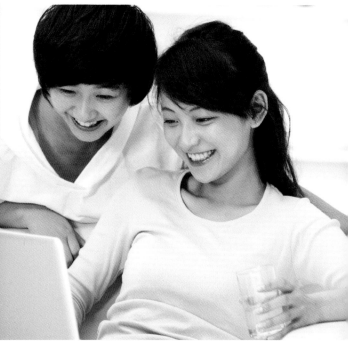

Lawrence Palevsky MD, Esther Park, Kyong Parker, Laurence Rosen MD, Lori Rothbard, Kathi Rota-Tebb, Orly Rumberg, Denise Schwendeman, Leticia Skelton, Arturo Soza, Kerry Stonehouse, Lupe Rivera, Guitty Roustai, Lisa Ullman, & Lorinda Walker.

Our publisher Life Science Publishing: especially Troie Battles and her traveling team: Jason Dang, Jason Jensen, Jeffrey Jensen, Matt Mackay, and Shauna Stout and everyone back at the office who are our "face" in the field. You've made this last year a lot of fun as we've started on this new adventure with your generous support. Paul Springer's great designs for all the YL90 products make the printed word come alive.

Our inspiration: D. Gary Young, a pioneer and tireless visionary.

Our followers on Facebook & Twitter, thank you for spreading the word!

And our friends from our Circle of the Work who pray for us daily.

We could not have done this without you. We love and thank you all.

In good health and deepest gratitude,
—*Carrie & Elena*

Introduction

Many people use essential oils; young and old alike. Before beginning this or any nutritional or exercise regimen consult your physician to be sure it is appropriate for you. To use your oils as safely as possible, please follow the guidelines below.

· ·

Essential oil and product guidelines:

1 Always consult a medical professional before you incorporate essential oils and supplements into your health regimen.

2 Never put an oil directly into the eyes or the ears. If you do get an essential oil into the eyes or ears, do not panic. Apply either V6 Mixing Oil or another fatty oil like olive oil with a soft cloth and gently wipe the essential oil out of the eyes. Within moments you should feel relief. If you have dripped an essential oil into the ear, you may pour a small amount of either V6 Mixing Oil or another fatty oil like olive oil into the ear and then tip the head to pour it out. This should remove any discomfort to the ear.

3 We prefer and trust Young Living Therapeutic-Grade Essential Oils. We believe that oils which are not safe enough to ingest should not be diffused into the air nor applied to the skin. Other commercial blends exist on the market but we find these blends to be superior in synergy, potency, and purity. The essential oil blend, supplement and personal product names used throughout are trademarks of Young Living Essential Oils.

4 Do not mix essential oils with synthetic personal care products, preservatives, or other adulterated foods.

5 Keep bottles closed, out of direct light and high heat, to keep your oils potent for many years.

6 Keep essential oils out of reach of small children.

7 Pregnant women should always use essential oils under the advisement of a medical professional.

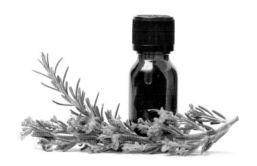

Now that you know how to use essential oils safely, how do you begin?

This book: *Essential Oils 101* is a beginner's guide. Here we have chosen products that we feel will help you get started using essential oils and products both quickly and easily. Once you have started you may want to try other products and learn more, so we've also provided you with a list of additional resources for each health issue.

The YL90™ Plan was developed by Carrie & Elena and is short for "Your Life in 90 Days". Our 90-day plans are found in the *YL90 Plan* brochures, books, magazines, iPhone & iPad App, and websites. It is a way to help you get healthy in 90 days using natural essential oils and products. It can also be found on Twitter, Facebook, MeetUp.com, and other social media. These are just some of the resources we provide to help you set out on the road to excellent natural health.

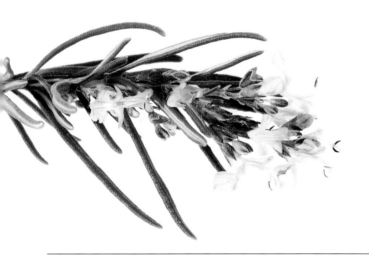

Let's get started:

1 Pick one of the 50 challenges listed here in *Essential Oils 101*. Taking on too many challenges at once is more difficult than dealing with them one at time.

2 Look at the suggested "Shopping List" for each challenge. Choose the products you are ready to try and commit to using them for at least 90 days.

3 Try a *YL90 Plan* for each challenge. There are YL90 plans to correspond with each of the challenges in the book which can provide additional support and information. You will see a picture of the suggested YL90 Plan brochure at the bottom of each left-hand page for every ailment.

4 The best way to order the products you need is through a regular monthly rewards program.

5 Remember you can support your health in three ways: applying, ingesting, and/or diffusing essential oils.

6 Share your results with others. See our tips to "Share with friends" that begins below.

7 Keep using your oils and supplements for daily support and as challenges arise. Carry your oils with you or put them where you are most likely to see and use them.

Share with friends:

When you find something that really works the first instinct is to share it...a great restaurant, movie, or a fun store! We are programed to pass things on. This sounds like an easy thing to do, but many people find that sharing can be challenging or even debilitating.

How do I share? With whom do I share? Will people reject my information? What if I don't communicate it well? What if I forget something? Sometimes these questions alone can stop someone from helping a family member or friend.

Essential Oils 101 and the *YL90 Plan* are the perfect tools for sharing. You don't need to remember or know anything to share successfully. These tools will do the work for you. Inexpensive and easy to understand, you can give both of these tools to a new or existing user. The information inside each brochure will help them try new things, apply oils to new situations, and give them the success story they need to begin sharing themselves.

One can't whip cream by blowing in a bowl, you need the right tool...a mixer or whisk. One also can't share essential oils and products without a tool. *Essential Oils 101* and the *YL90* plans are the perfect tools to help you get started; fast, easy, and effective.

Follow these easy steps:

1   Carry a copy of *Essential Oils 101* wherever you go. Get extra copies and share them with your friends, colleagues, family members, and others you meet.

2   Listen. If someone expresses a need that *Essential Oils 101* can support, offer them information in this book. Each suggestion in this book is easy to get, easy to follow, and easy to share.

3   Plan your work for the next 3 months; "Meeting-in-a-Box" makes this easy.

4   Hold a YL90 Plan meeting using a "Meeting-in-a-Box." Follow your brochure. Don't over-talk, over-explain, provide too much "science," argue with naysayers, or attempt to convince people of anything!

5   Go to www.YL90Plan.com, or better yet, send a friend there, too. At our website you will find podcasts, a blog, videos, and lots of other FREE information. You can sign up for Facebook and "LIKE" our page at www.facebook.com/getaplan to join our growing chat group of other like-minded essential oil users sharing information for free.

Here's to your good health!
Enjoy the book.

—Carrie & Elena

. . . .

Suggested Reading

Permission Marketing: Turning Strangers Into Friends And Friends Into Customers by Seth Godin (Hardcover, May 6, 1999)

The Back of the Napkin (Expanded Edition): *Solving Problems and Selling Ideas with Pictures* by Dan Roam (Hardcover, Dec 31, 2009)

Delivering Happiness: A Path to Profits, Passion, and Purpose by Tony Hsieh (Hardcover, Jun 7, 2010)

Essential Oils Business Book - How to Start, Build, and Prosper in the Essential Oil Industry by Christina Calisto-Winslow (Paperback, June 1, 2010)

Your Mother Was Right: All the Great Advice You Tried to Forget by Kate Reardon (Paperback, Aug. 3, 2010)

Addiction & Substance Abuse

Addiction & Substance Abuse is a physical or psychological dependence on something for which you feel no control. Many substances cross the blood-brain barrier altering the chemical environment of the brain.

. . . .

Tip: Do not try to do this alone. Support is critical to overcoming addictions. Find a buddy to help you order, use your products, and stick to your program. You can do this!

. . . .

Our Approach:

Apply: *JuvaCleanse* over the liver and on the bottom of the feet 2 times daily. Drink plenty of water while using your oils to flush all toxins from the body.

Try: 1 one drop of *Clove* and one drop of *Dill* to the tip of the tongue every time a craving occurs. *Peppermint* has been known to reduce food addictions when used very frequently throughout the day.

Cleansing: is core to addiction cessation. Incorporate the *Cleansing Trio* to your daily routine. You may have to use the *Cleansing Trio* for a year or more to clear your body of its addiction.

Diffuse: *Inspiration*, *Abundance*, or *Surrender* blends to change the chemical environment of your brain so that you can maintain your sobriety.

Note: If addictions run in your family be proactive. Talk to your children to increase awareness of what they may have to face and incorporate cleansing at a young age. If enzymes and cleansing oils are part of daily life, toxins which lead to addiction have a harder time taking hold. Find a positive substitute for the addictive substance. A runner's high is a great alternative to chocolate cake or alcohol.

If your suffer from depression, in addition to an addiction, your struggle may be 10 times worse. Dealing with the depression can unlock the strength you need to overcome your addictions. Going on depression medications can lead to other addictions and may not be the most desirable course. Try following the YL90 Plan called *End the Blues*. This plan can be used by persons of all ages and includes nutritional and essential oil therapy.

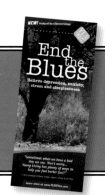

Dear Carrie & Elena,

Over the last few years I had several family challenges that led me to unhealthy eating to deal with stress. As my life began to change in a positive direction the one habit I found the most difficult to stop was drinking too much orange soda pop. My mouth would water when I would see the can! And I was drinking up to a 6-pack a day. My daughter-in-law told me about Dill oil. I thought it sounded goofy, but I was willing to try anything. She said to try it on my wrists. I put it on every day like perfume and it smelled good. Slowly but surely the craving diminished, it took a few months, but I wanted less soda and finally I didn't want any at all. My daughter-in-law also said a drop on the tongue works well too, but I never needed it. Of course, when I stopped drinking so much soda, my weight dropped too. I feel a lot healthier.

— Dahlia R. NY

SINGLES:

Clove
Dill
Peppermint

OIL BLENDS:

Abundance
Inspiration
JuvaCleanse
Surrender

SUPPLEMENTS:

Cleansing Trio

Did You Know?

If you suffer from addiction you are not alone. Of the American population, 27% suffer from an addiction or substance abuse. This has a critical effect on the health of our society with more than 40% of traffic deaths and 50% of homicides being related to addiction at a cost to society of $414 billion in 2009. Needless to say, freeing yourself from an addiction is life changing.

"The chains of habit are generally too small to be felt until they are too strong to be broken."

—Samuel Johnson—

| **Suggested Reading** | *Cures for Modern Times* by Journey Editions. Includes *The Hangover Pack,* which includes Almond Oil and Lavender and Rosemary Essential Oils (Paperback, Mar. 1997) | *Guide to Tobacco Freedom with Aromatherapy* by Audrey Benenati (Kindle Edition - Kindle eBook, Dec. 1, 2009) |

Allergies

Allergies can be caused by: hay fever, seasonal changes, poison ivy & plants, molds, foods, animals, insect bites, drugs, cosmetics, & cleaners.

· · · · · · ·

Tip: When coming back from a baseball game or other outdoor activity, remove clothing immediately and put aside for washing. Take a shower to remove pollen that may have settled on skin and hair.

· · · · · · ·

Our Approach:

Apply: *Breathe Again Roll-on* along the sides of the nose, down the throat, and on the back of the neck to help relieve symptoms. Apply *Tranquil Roll-on* around a rash to sooth the itch.

Try: Drinking 1 oz. of *NingXia Red* with 1 full capsule of *Lavender* 2-4 times a day. Add 2 drops of *Roman Chamomile* to the *Lavender* capsule if symptoms persist.

Diffuse: *Lavender* at night, and *RC* during the day, to support normal respiration.

Did you know?

Allergies have been long thought of as a chronic condition something that cannot be "undone." If the body can be weakened, why can it not be strengthened?

Our experiences with the allergies of our family and friends has shown that a dedication to an oil and supplement program designed to strengthen the bodies defenses against allergies can help. We like to start using our allergy oils at least one month before our allergies usually strike. This proactive approach may help to lessen the severity of your allergy season or allow you to skip it entirely!

If your allergies are seasonal, for example, begin the YL90 Plan: *Live Free of Allergies, Asthma, Eczema* one month after allergy season has ended.

Providing your body with good nutritional support may just be what your body needs to keep you symptom free. Continue following the YL90 Plan through the season. Maybe next year you can use less or even find your allergies don't come back!

Dear Carrie & Elena,

I have had severe seasonal allergies since childhood. Last year was particularly bad. Runny nose, fatigue, hives--you name it. I started taking 5 drops of lavender in a capsule along with a shot of NingXia Red (one ounce) twice daily. The symptoms went away in 2 days, and now I just use as needed. I have not taken an allergy pill since. When I get symptoms now, which are rare, I just take a lavender capsule and NingXia Red and I am fine. No side effects either; a much better plan for me.

— Donna M., NJ

OIL BLENDS:
Breathe Again Roll-on
Tranquil Roll-on
RC

SINGLES:
Lavender
Roman Chamomile

SUPPLEMENTS:
NingXia Red

OTHER:
Vegetable Capsules

I used to wake up at 4 A.M. and start sneezing, sometimes for five hours. I tried to find out what sort of allergy I had but finally came to the conclusion that it must be an allergy to consciousness.

—James Thurber—

| **Suggested Reading** | *The Whole Soy Story: The Dark Side of America's Favorite Health Food* by Kaayla T. Daniel (Hardcover, Mar. 10, 2005) | *Natural Home Health Care Using Essential Oils* by Daniel Pénoël, M.D. (Paperback, Aug. 1998) |

Alzheimer's & Dementia

Alzheimer's is the most common form of dementia, a general term for loss of memory and other intellectual abilities serious enough to interfere with daily life. Alzheimer's disease accounts for 50 to 80 percent of all dementia cases. Parkinson's disease, and other issues that effect the central nervous system are often classified with dementia.

. . . .

Tip: If your loved one suffers from irritability, try applying calming oils to the temples or feet while they are sleeping to improve their waking mood.

. . . .

Our Approach:

Apply: *Sacred Frankincense* to the back of the neck often through the day. Apply **Brain Power** to the big toes and **Clarity** to the temples in the morning.

Try: Three to nine **OmegaGize** capsules a day and 1 packet of **True Source** vitamins for nutritional support.

Diffuse: *Frankincense* at night, and **Peace & Calming** during the day to promote relaxation.

Did you know?

The silent invasion of Alzheimer's and dementia can take a physically healthy loved one and mentally and emotionally remove them from their life as they know it.

The effects of physically connecting with your loved one during the process of applying oils may help to improve their quality of life. "Touch is the first language we learn," according to University of California, Berkeley, Psychologist Dacher Keltner and is a powerful healing tool. In a world where drug therapy has often fallen short, the basic healing practice of touch with essential oils has made great strides in improving quality of life without bringing on unwanted side effects.

Depression and anxiety can affect those suffering from Alzheimer's and dementia as well as their friends and families. Being on a wellness program that supports a positive mood can help you and your loved one to deal with the challenges you face.

The YL90 Plan, *End the Blues*, incorporates both a nutritional program and an oils program that can be used together or separately to lift the spirit!

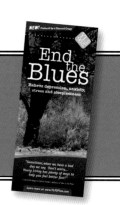

Dear Carrie & Elena,

At only 51 years old I was diagnosed with Parkinson's Disease. I started by drinking 4 to 6 oz. of NingXia Red daily. I was pleasantly surprised that I felt the effect of the NingXia Red almost immediately. I had more energy and was able to get through each day without napping as much.

Next, using the Neuro-Auricular Technique, originated by Gary Young. My wife applied Frankincense, Valerian, Vetiver, Roman Chamomile, Cedarwood, & Sandalwood daily. We start with the Frankincense at the base of my skull and then continue the oils in the order listed above applied one at a time to about the middle of my spine. A couple of months later I added a drop of Melissa under my tongue daily, plus Core Supplements, BLM, and Sulfurzyme.

The result of this regimen is that I have more energy, I'm now able to do my physical therapy which increases my mobility plus I've been able to lower my prescribed medications. The side effects that I was experiencing with the medications such as sleep apnea and cognitive confusion have diminished as the medications have been lowered. I currently have substantially more energy and consistent mobility of the entire right side of my body. I feel better than I have in three years!

— Al G., OH

Faced with explaining Alzheimer's to her own children, Maria Shriver said "I wrote a book called, What's Happening to Grandpa? At the time, I said I wrote it to help my children understand what was happening. In truth, I wrote it to explain Alzheimer's to myself."

Suggested Reading   *Aromatherapy for Healing the Spirit: Restoring Emotional and Mental Balance with Essential Oils* by Gabriel Mojay (Jan 1, 2000)

Aromatherapy: Soothing Remedies to Restore, Rejuvenate and Heal by Valerie Gennari Cooksley (May 30, 2002)

Asthma

Asthma is a chronic, inflammatory lung disease involving recurrent breathing problems. Asthma affects more than 17 million people in the United States and a third of these are children. Asthma affects people of all races and is slightly more common in African Americans.

(National Institute of Allergy and Infectious Disease)

Tip: Part of lessening an asthma attack is being able to stay calm. Incorporating deep breathing exercises not only strengthens the lungs but calms the spirit.

Our Approach:

Apply: *Eucalyptus Blue* and *Breathe Again Roll-on* liberally to chest, back, and bottom of the feet morning and night.

Try: One ounce of *NingXia Red* with 2 drops of *Frankincense*, and 2 drops of *Lemon* 2-4 times a day to support the respiratory system.

Diffuse: Rotating between the 3 oils *RC*, *Raven* and *Hyssop*, 15 minutes per day, to promote normal respiration. If you are experiencing an asthma attack, seek medical attention!

Did you know?

Asthma can be scary. Not knowing when an attack will strike can put the asthma sufferer in a constant state of concern; even panic. This stress can not only bring on an asthma attack, it can worsen an attack when triggered.

Try using relaxing essential oils. Carry *Stress Away Roll-on* during the day and apply *Peace & Calming*, *Tranquil Roll-on*, or *RutaVaLa* to your feet nightly to help balance your stress and fortify your body against an asthma attack. Once asthma strikes, you may not be able to breathe in these oils so be proactive by applying oils to the feet when your asthma is under control.

In addition to the YL90 Plan: *Live Free of Allergies, Asthma, & Eczema* follow the recipes in our *Green Your Body, Green Your Home* brochure.

Researcher Jan-Paul Zock, PhD, found that "Asthma increased with the frequency of use and the number of different (cleaning) products used, with a 30% to 50% increase in asthma risk. As many as one in seven asthma cases in adults may be caused by the use of spray cleaners."

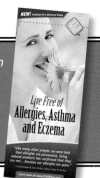

Live Free of
**Allergies, Asthma
and Eczema**

Dear Carrie & Elena,

I have suffered from severe allergic, asthmatic bronchitis since 1981. I used 2 inhalers, an antihistamine (sometimes doubling the dosage per doctor's orders) and Singulair. Some seasons would be so bad that I would also need a dose of Prednisone to start and allow me to just breath. Well, in November of 2009 I started using essential oils. I would put 2 drops of Frankincense on my crown morning and Breath Again Roll-on on my chest morning and night. I have not used any inhalers since March 2010, nor have I had an asthma attack since!

For the allergies, I drink 1-2 oz. of NingXia Red daily and either 2 drops of Lavender in my NingXia Red or if it's a bad allergy season (like this one is) I will take a full capsule of Lavender in the morning with my 1 oz. of NingXia Red. I have not taken an antihistamine since March 2010 nor have I taken any Singulair since then. I am able to enjoy the outdoors and not get bronchitis or laryngitis. I can be around flowers without suffering unmercifully. No itchy, watery eyes and runny nose or sneezing!

— LindaSue A., NJ

Shopping List

SINGLES:
Eucalyptus blue
Frankincense
Hyssop
Lavender
Lemon

OIL BLENDS:
Breathe Again Roll-on
Peace & Calming
Raven
RC
RutaVaLa Roll-on
Tranquil Roll-on

SUPPLEMENTS:
NingXia Red

Suggested Reading

Essential Oils Desk Reference by Life Science Publishing (NEW 2011 5th edition)

Coil Bound *Quick Reference Guide for Using Essential Oils* by Connie and Alan Higley (New 12th Edition, July 2010 Revision)

The Essential Oils Handbook: All the Oils You Will Ever Need for Health, Vitality and Well-Being by Jennie Harding (Paperback, Jun 3, 2008)

Autoimmune Disease Support

Autoimmune disease causes the body's protective force to attack itself. The name of the disease depends upon the location of the organ under attack. There are more than 100 known autoimmune diseases in the world today and the list is growing.

. . . .

Tip: Consider cleansing part of your daily routine to help control inflammation. Drinking *NingXia Red* daily or taking *Essential*zyme capsules at night are two ways to promote daily gentle cleansing.

. . . .

Our Approach:

Apply: *Regenolone* and *PanAway* to help reduce body aches, *Thieves* blend to the bottom of the feet to support immunity, and carry *Deep Relief Roll-on* during the day to apply essential oils easily if pain strikes.

Try: 1 drop of *Melissa* under the tongue 2-4 times a day. Drink 2 oz. of *NingXia Red* 3 times a day. Take *Core Supplements* and drink a *Balance Complete* shake to support good nutrition. Try **PD 80/20** capsules to support endocrine balance.

Diffuse: *Peppermint* during the day and *Peace & Calming* at night.

Did you know?

This topic is very close to my heart as my mother has suffered from Lupus for more than 50 years. I know that when the disease is at its most virulent, your energy level can plummet. In addition to the pain and suffering endured, patients also have to contend with physical exhaustion.

Bringing up your energy level can be almost as beneficial as putting the disease in remission. Applying 2 drops of *En-R-Gee* to the back of the neck, drinking 4 oz. daily of *NingXia Red*, and taking *Super B* tablets can help to bring up your energy for as much as 4 hours at a time helping you to feel "normal" again.

The Raindrop Technique™ massage has been found to be very supportive when managing autoimmune disease. While, finding a Raindrop Technique practitioner in your area is ideal, you can do it yourself by following the video contained in every Raindrop Oils Kit.

Incorporating the nutritional plan in the YL90 Plan brochure, *Who Needs a Raindrop? Everyone!* is an easy way to support the nutritional needs of someone with an autoimmune disease.

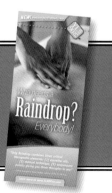

Dear Carrie & Elena,

I live with Crohn's Autoimmune Disorder... Frankincense along with NingXia Red has allowed me to be prescription drug free for the first time in years.

— Heather F., OH

Every human being is the author of his own health or disease.

—Buddha—

Suggested Reading

What Your Doctor May Not Tell You About Autoimmune Disorders: The Revolutionary, Drug-Free Treatments for Thyroid Disease, Lupus, MS, IBD, Chronic Fatigue; Rheumatoid Arthritis, and Other Diseases by Stephen B. Edelson and Deborah Mitchell (Paperback, Mar. 2003)

Medical Aromatherapy: Healing with Essential Oils by Kurt Schnaubelt (Jan 12, 1999)

The Complete Book of Enzyme Therapy: A Complete and Up-to-Date Reference to Effective Remedies by Anthony J. Cichoke (Nov 15, 1998)

Blood Pressure

About 1 in 3 adults in the United States has High Blood Pressure (HBP). The condition itself frequently has no symptoms and you can have it for years without knowing it. This "silent" condition, HBP, can damage the heart, blood vessels, kidneys, and other parts of your body.

Our Approach:

Apply: One to two drops of *Aroma Life* and *Peace & Calming* over the heart.

Try: A *Power Meal* shake as a meal substitute, which may help to balance blood pressure.

Diffuse: *Ylang Ylang* or *Peace & Calming* to clear the mind and reduce pressure and stress.

Did You Know?

Dealing with stress is key to maintaining healthy blood pressure. If you struggle with stress in your life pick one task in your day that you can eliminate. Taking on too much can lead to serious health risks.

Trying to lose weight to decrease your blood pressure? Instead of sharing a meal with a friend ask them to help you with a fun or mundane task around your house or an errand you have to run. This will give you "face time" with your friend while checking something off your "to do" list freeing up some time for yourself and avoiding the high-fat trap of restaurant food. Managing work and tasks with others reduces stress. Incorporate stress-reducing oils like: *Stress Away Roll-on*, *Valor*, and *Peace & Calming* to help your blood pressure stay in a healthy range.

Being overweight or obese increases your risk of developing high blood pressure. In fact, your blood pressure rises as your body weight increases. Losing even 10 pounds can lower your blood pressure—and losing weight has the biggest effect on those who are overweight and already have hypertension. (National Institutes of Health)

Try our easy program in the brochure, *Fat Loss that Works!* Our program gives you a weight loss guide for foods, oils, and supplements.

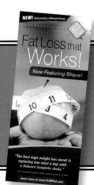

Shopping List

SINGLES:
Ylang Ylang

OIL BLENDS:
Aroma Life
Peace & Calming
Stress Away Roll-on
Valor

SUPPLEMENTS:
Power Meal

Dear Carrie & Elena,

I took my blood pressure monitor one day and tested several oils that are said to lower blood pressure. I recorded the reading, then waited 10 minutes and took it again while inhaling an oil.

I did this over several days with several oils and found the results were remarkable in lowering my blood pressure. Lavender actually lowered it by almost 20 points! Aroma Life, Goldenrod, Ylang Ylang, Clove, Lemon, and Marjoram were also very effective.

Now my husband & I are both off meds and just take a drop or two of Lavender daily to keep our blood pressure within perfectly normal limits.

— Leticia S., NJ

"One way to get high blood pressure is to go mountain climbing over molehills."

—Earl Wilson—

Tip: Loading up on potassium-rich fruits and vegetables is an important part of any blood pressure–lowering program. Aim for potassium levels of up to 4,000 mg a day, says Linda Van Horn, PhD, RD, professor of preventive medicine at University Feinberg School of Medicine.

Suggested Reading

Lower Your Blood Pressure in Eight Weeks: A Revolutionary Program for a Longer, Healthier Life by Stephen T. Sinatra (Feb 4, 2003)

Aromatherapy for Dummies by Kathi Keville (Paperback, Sept. 15, 1999)

Reversing Heart Disease: A Vital New Program to Help Prevent, Treat, and Eliminate Cardiac Problems Without Surgery by Julian M. Whitaker (Paperback - Mar. 1, 2002)

Brain Power

When you feel foggy, forgetful, or scattered, it may be time to feed your brain. The brain, made up mostly of fat, will perform at its highest level when we fed. Our brain not only controls how we think but also how the rest of our body's systems perform.

....

Tip: Studies show that students who study late at night on caffeine find their short-term memory fails them on the next day's exam. (January 2009 issue of Behavioral Sleep Medicine)

Skip the coffee and take a shot or 2 of **NingXia Red** and 4 **Multigreens** capsules. You can repeat this every 4 hours.

....

Apply: A few drops of **Brain Power** to the big toes and **Sacred Frankincense**, **Valor**, **Stress Away Roll-on**, and **RutaVala Roll-on** to the spine. Apply **Helichrysum** to the brain stem to support the CNS (central nervous system).

Try: **OmegaGize** & **Longevity** capsules 1-2 times daily. If you have trouble sleeping, try taking 1-2 **Sleepessence** capsules. **Essentialzyme** capsules can help with digestion and nutrient assimilation; a healthy body yields a healthy brain.

Diffuse: **Cedarwood** day and night. You can also add **Lavender** or **Peace & Calming** to help you sleep more soundly at night.

Dear Carrie & Elena,

My autistic 11 year old is off ALL prescription medication (that have to do with his autistic symptoms) thanks to BrainPower, Valor and Cedarwood! He will ask for more if and when his body needs it during homework time or if he is nervous before school!

— Heather K., OH.

There are many everyday chemicals we use without understanding their effect on our bodies. Fluoride, found in most toothpastes, has been shown to be toxic to several body systems. —Robert J. Carton and J. William Hirzy, EPA. Switching to the Thieves line of toothpastes is an easy way to eliminate a common toxin.

The YL90 Plan brochure, *Green Cleaning Solutions* will teach you how to remove dangerous chemical cleaners and personal care products and replace them with natural alternatives.

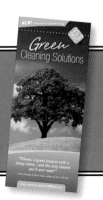

*Genius is seeing what everyone else sees and
thinking what no-one else has thought.*

—Albert Szent-Gyorgy, scientist, discovered Vitamin C—

•••➤

Did you know?

ADD/ADHD is becoming more and more prevalent. Although the causes are
controversial, regular exercise can help such as: walking or riding a bike.
Getting enough sleep is also critical. Start your bed time routine early with
calming oils and no electronics to ensure a healthy amount of sleep. Include
supplements rich in fish oils like **OmegaGize**.

Another troubling ailment that effects the brain is autism. Consider adding
enzymes to your diet. Taken before meals, enzymes are effective at improving
symptoms such as attention deficit, socialization, hyperactivity, eye contact,
comprehension and compulsions,

—Timothy Buie, MD, Pediatric Gastroenterology, Harvard/Mass General Hospital.

The aromas from therapeutic essential oils have a powerful ability to stimulate
the limbic region of the brain, because the sense of smell is tied directly to the
mind's emotional and hormonal centers. As a result, the aroma of an essential
oil has the potential to exert a powerful influence on ADD/ADHD and Autism.

— Dr. Terry Friedmann, MD

> ## Shopping List
>
> ### SINGLES:
> *Cedarwood*
> *Helichrysum*
> *Lavender*
> *Sacred Frankincense*
>
> ### OIL BLENDS:
> *Brain Power*
> *Peace & Calming*
> *RutaVaLa*
> *Stress Away Roll-on*
> *Valor*
>
> ### SUPPLEMENTS:
> *Essentialzyme*
> *Longevity*
> *Multigreens*
> *NingXia Red*
> *OmegaGize*
> *Sleepessence*

| Suggested Reading | *The Better Brain Book* by David Perlmutter, M.D., FACN (Paperback, Aug. 2, 2005) | *Vaccines: The Risks, the Benefits, the Choices, a Resource Guide for Parents* by Sherri J. Tenpenny (Paperback, Jan. 1, 2006) | *The A.D.D. and A.D.H.D. Diet!* by Rachel Bell and Dr. Howard Peiper (Paperback, June 5, 2004) |

Breast Health

Know your breasts. Changes in breast shape, size, & feel are common and many changes are benign. Conduct regular self-breast examinations and stay in close contact with your doctor about your breast health so that you can detect problems as early as possible.

. . . .

Tip: Cancers feed on sugar. Limiting your intake of sugars can significantly reduce your risk of breast cancers. Taking **Essentialzyme** daily will help you process the sugars you do eat more effectively.

. . . .

Our Approach:

Apply: One to four drops of **Frankincense** daily to each breast and use 1-2 drops of **Progessence Plus** on a fatty tissue such as the hips, thighs, & belly.

Try: *Core Supplements* vitamins and drink 2 ounces **NingXia Red** daily.

Diffuse: *Lavender* at night to promote good sleep and healthy cell regeneration.

Did you know?

You can make a date with yourself for breast health! Every October (during Breast Cancer Awareness Month) and April (6 months later) use Gary Young's program for breast health.

Apply **Frankincense**, **Tsuga**, **Myrtle**, & **Sandalwood** to the breasts every day for the entire month. (Dilute with organic olive oil if you experience any discomfort.) Use up all 4 bottles by the end of the month. Be generous: this is the best gift you can give yourself, a friend, or sister!

Take **Orange** oil in capsules during the month, also using up the bottle (about 5-6 drops per day).

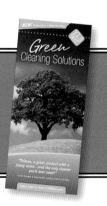

Are household cleaners linked to breast cancer? In a study published recently in the *Journal of Environmental Health*, breast cancer risk was highest among women who reported the greatest use of cleaning products and air fresheners. The risk was twice that of those who reported low use of these products.

Use the natural products found in the YL90 Plan brochure, *Green Cleaning Solutions* to get started!

Dear Carrie & Elena,

Every January I try to get away from the cold weather and take a trip to Florida. Before I left last year I had a mammogram. My mammograms had always been normal (I am 80 years old). This time the doctor told me they saw a small spot, but not to worry (ha, ha, ha). I was leaving for my trip the next day and not sure what to do.

I decided to go away anyway and apply Frankincense oil, diluted, with V6 Mixing Oil to my breasts every day. I also took one full capsule of Orange oil in the morning and evening and I put myself in God's hands.

During my month away I spent lots of time relaxing in fresh sea air with my friends. When I got back, I had a follow-up mammogram and both the technician and the doctor were amazed to see that there was nothing there. I, of course, was greatly relieved.

— Clara O., NY

Shopping List

SINGLES:

Frankincense
Lavender
Myrtle
Orange
Sandalwood
Tsuga

SUPPLEMENTS:

Core Supplements
Essentialzyme
NingXia Red

PERSONAL CARE:

Progessence Plus

"You gain strength, courage and confidence by every experience in which you really stop to look fear in the face."

—Eleanor Roosevelt—

Suggested Reading *Dr. Susan Love's Breast Book*, 5th Edition (A Merloyd Lawrence Book) by Susan M. Love MD and Karen Lindsey (Sep 14, 2010)

What Your Doctor May Not Tell You About Breast Cancer by John R. Lee, M.D., David Zava, Ph.D., and Virginia Hopkins (Paperback, Mar. 1, 2005)

Bug Bites & Repellents

Bugs can transmit diseases to you and your pets and although not every bite is toxic, it is certainly best to avoid them as they are generally uncomfortable. If you are bitten, be sure to find out what bit you and if necessary have it tested.

· · · · · · ·

Tip: To repel pests, apply an essential oil such as **Cedarwood** (or other type of conifer oil). Give special attention to the warmest, leanest parts of your body—neck, armpits, ears, wrists—wherever blood vessels are close to the surface.

· · · · · · ·

Our Approach:

Apply: *Purification* to the bite to reduce swelling and draw out any infection. Apply **PanAway** around the bite to reduce pain and inflammation. Repeat as needed.

Try: An **Inner Defense** capsule each day for a week after being bitten. Drink 1 oz. of **NingXia Red** & take 1 **Longevity** capsule to help keep your immune system strong.

Diffuse: *Purification* to help keep bugs from coming back!

Did you know?

We have travelled all over the world, and no matter where you go there are always bugs. Eating the foods of the region and avoiding sugars is one way to keep bugs at bay. You want to smell like a local!

Taking oils internally that repel bugs, like **Peppermint**, can also help keep pests away as the oils begin to perspire from your pores. If you are bitten or stung roll on **Tranquil Roll-on** around the bite. The 3 oils in **Tranquil Roll-on**: **Roman Chamomile**, **Lavender**, and **Cedarwood** act as an anti-histamine and may help to prevent an allergic reaction.

Don't just apply your oils once. Swimming and perspiration will diminish the effect of the oils. Apply often to provide the protection you need.

Sharing essential oils with others can be as simple as helping them keep the bugs away! Many essential oils are disliked by pests. We like to place cotton balls soaked in *Purification* around platters of food at a picnic — bugs stay away without harmful chemicals.

Follow the suggestions in the YL90 Plan brochure, *Enjoy The Great Outdoors*, and have a bug-free healthy summer!

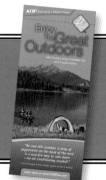

Dear Carrie & Elena,

I was sorting through a box of vegetables from a farmer's market one day and unexpectedly grabbed a bee that was hidden in the box! The sting was intense. I grabbed Purification and PanAway and watched as the swelling decreased, the pain subsided and after several applications of each, the bite was nearly gone by the end of the day!

—Lou L., OH

.... ➤

....

Shopping List

SINGLES:
Peppermint

OIL BLENDS:
PanAway
Purification
Tranquil Roll-on

SUPPLEMENTS:
Inner Defense
Longevity
NingXia Red

"I loved being outside. We'd hold lightning bugs in our fingers and pretend they were diamond rings."

—Loretta Lynn—

Suggested Reading	
Suggested Reading	_The One Gift_ by D. Gary Young (Hardcover - 2010)
	Aromatherapy for Dummies by Kathi Keville (Paperback, Sep 15, 1999)

Burns

There are 3 types of burns: first, second, and third degree burns. The first degree does not burn through the outer layer of skin, the second burns through only the first layer and, the third burns through all layers; skin, fat, and even at times bone. Be sure to know the type of burn you have. Burns should receive a proper diagnosis and immediate medical attention.

Our Approach:

Apply: *PanAway* around, never on, the affected area. To help with the pain, apply **Cypress** to the feet (not near the wound). **Lavaderm Spray** can be used every 20 minutes. Once the wound scabs over, apply **Frankincense**, **Helichrysum**, or **Lavender** topped with **Rose Ointment** for healing.

Try: Drink **NingXia Red**, and take **OmegaGize**, & **Sulfurzyme** capsules 2 times a day. Take 2 drops each of **Clove**, **Helichrysum**, **Vetiver**, & **Valerian** in a capsule to help minimize the pain. This may cause drowsiness so be sure to allow yourself time to rest.

Diffuse: *Peace & Calming*. A relaxed body heals faster.

Tip: Mild sunburns can be soothed with a spritz of **Lavaderm Spray**. **Lavaderm** contains aloe and lavender, two known skin healing agents. Wearing light clothes and a hat that covers your skin from the sun is the best protection. Sunscreen should be used sparingly. Foods with beta carotene like carrots and squash help to build natural sun protection in the skin.

"Holding on to anger is like grasping a hot coal with the intent of throwing it at someone else; you are the one who gets burned."

—Buddha—

Burns must be tended well to heal. Taking care of the skin--keeping it clean, protected, and free from infection is key. We like to keep *Melrose* around for burns. Whether from the sun or the stove, *Melrose* on your feet and around the burn will help to keep infection away.

Check out our other great tips in the YL90 Plan brochure, *The Great Outdoors*, and be prepared in case of an emergency.

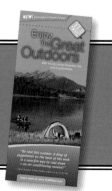

Dear Carrie & Elena,

I accidentally spilled a cup of boiling hot tea on my chest, lap, & legs. Challenged with a skin-healing disorder, no medications were able to help me. I sprayed on Lavaderm as often as every 20 minutes until my wounds were healed!

—Sally T., OH

Did you know?

Scars develop on the skin's surface as the result of burns, deep lacerations or a variety of other injuries that penetrate or interrupt the skin's integrity. The skin forms a scab over a wound within three to four days following an injury. By day ten the scab typically shrinks and sloughs off as the body focuses on laying down collagen fibers to strengthen the former site of injury. In cases of severe injury the damaged tissue can be in recovery for up to three months before it returns to full strength.

Gently massaging around the area will promote healing and diminish scarring. Only 15 minutes a day, can help the area get the proper circulation. Do not massage to the point of pain. Try massaging with a little **Frankincense**, **Lavender**, or **Helichrysum**. —Nicole Cutler, L.Ac.

Suggested Reading

Aroma: The International Magazine for Essential Oils. Nr. 1/Winter 2000: Lavender. by Terra Linda Scent and Image Inc. (Hardcover, 2000)

The Aromatherapy Encyclopedia, A Concise Guide to Over 385 Plant Oils by Carol Schiller (Paperback, Jun. 2008)

Cancer

Cancer takes on many different forms and symptoms. The steps below are for general health support to strengthen the body's defenses against cancer. The recommendations are good for those who want to prevent, are addressing, or are recovering from cancer. As always, all natural products should be used under the advisement of your health care practitioner.

Our Approach:

Apply: Four drops of any of the following oils: *Frankincense, Orange, Lavender, Thyme, Myrrh, Lemongrass, Sandalwood, Tsuga, Clove* to your feet or along the spine. Dilute if the skin is sensitive.

Try: Drinking **NingXia Red**, 2 oz. at a time, up to 8 oz. total per day; taking **Core Supplements**, **Essentialzyme** capsules and **Alkalime** before each meal; and taking a ½ capsule of **Orange** oil 2 times daily.

Diffuse: *Lavender* or *Valor* to reduce stress.

Tip: Ginger root contains compounds that may help relieve or prevent nausea and vomiting. These substances can increase the flow of saliva and digestive juices. They may also help to calm the stomach and intestines.

A 2009 Stanford University School of Medicine study found a link between cancer recurrence and early death in patients who also suffer from depression.

Fortify your health with products to support your mood. The YL90 Plan: *End the Blues* will give you a program of oils and supplements to keep your spirits high during times of struggle and challenge. This program is also helpful for those supporting a loved one with cancer.

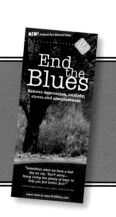

Dear Carrie & Elena,

After chemotherapy treatment for Acute Myelegenous Leukemia (AML) our son developed a fungal infection in his lung. With a very diminished immune system it's difficult to fight off the possible havoc to his body this fungal infection could wreak.

Another added worry was that without clearing the infection he would not have been able to receive a bone marrow transplant that he needed to remain cancer free in the future.

He was taking an anti–fungal medication as well as an antibiotic but we felt we needed to be more proactive. We simply could not wait to see if the medications would work and we began thinking of oils that we knew were combative to fungal infections.

We immediately started our son on a program of Melaleuca Alternifolia, Oregano & Thyme. We layered all three oils on the Vita Flex points on his feet every two hours while he was awake for three full weeks. We also diffused Melaleuca Alternifolia for a half hour -three times a day. Diffusing the Melaleuca Alternifolia at night lessened his congestion and coughing so he was able to fall asleep much easier.

The scans of his lungs taken after three weeks showed significant improvement to the point where the doctors commented on how well he was responding to the anti-fungal!

A small pocket of the fungal infection did have to be surgically removed but this outcome was significantly better than the original diagnosis!

Throughout the entire bone marrow transplant process we kept him well out of danger from a raging fungal infection by diffusing and applying the oils as we had above.

We know that the oils gave us an incredible advantage in this battle, a battle that many have lost. There was something so magical and healing for us to be able to lovingly apply the essential oils to our son with the intention of assisting him back to good health. Three years later and our entire family continues to use Young Living essential oils and supplements and are grateful to have them in our lives.

—Anonymous

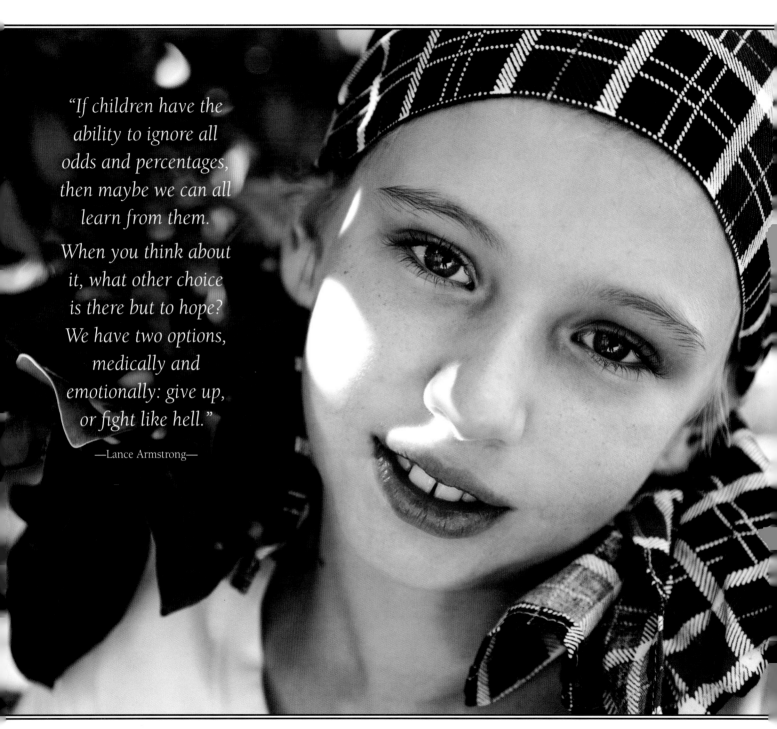

"If children have the ability to ignore all odds and percentages, then maybe we can all learn from them.

When you think about it, what other choice is there but to hope? We have two options, medically and emotionally: give up, or fight like hell."

—Lance Armstrong—

Did you know?

There are essential oils and essential oil-based products that can help with symptom relief:

- Anxiety: **Valor** and **Stress Away Roll-on** (on the pulse points)

- Dry Skin: **Genesis Lotion** (for the whole body)

- Exhaustion: **En-R-Gee** (on the nape of the neck)

- Hair Loss: **Lavender Mint Shampoo & Conditioner** (for safe, gentle cleaning)

- Insomnia: **ImmuPro** chewable tablets or **Sleepessence** capsules

- Mouth sores: **Thieves toothpastes and Thieves Mouthwash** (for gentle non-toxic cleaning)

- Nausea: **Ginger** or **Peppermint** (a drop on the tongue or diffuse)

- Pain: **PanAway** (at the site of pain or around if there is a wound)

Shopping List

SINGLES:
Clove
Frankincense
Ginger
Lavender
Lemongrass
Orange
Myrrh
Peppermint
Sandalwood
Thyme
Tsuga

OIL BLENDS
En-R-Gee
PanAway
Stress Away Roll-on
Valor

SUPPLEMENTS:
Alkalime
Core Supplements
Essentialzyme
ImmuPro
NingXia Red
Sleepessence

PERSONAL CARE:
Thieves Toothpaste
Genesis Lotion
Lavender Mint Conditioner
Lavender Mint Shampoo
Thieves Mouthwash

Suggested Reading

A More Excellent Way w/ DVD by Henry Wright (Apr 7, 2009)

Heal Your Body by Louise L. Hay (Paperback, 1998)

Encyclopedia of Natural Medicine, Revised Second Edition by Michael Murray and Joseph Pizzorno (Dec 29, 1997)

Aromatherapy for Health Professionals by Len Price Cert Ed MIT(Trichology) FISPA FIAM and Shirley Price Cert Ed FISPA MIFA FIAM (Dec 5, 2006)

Medical Aromatherapy: Healing with Essential Oils by Kurt Schnaubelt (Jan 12, 1999)

Candida & Yeast Infection

Candida and yeast are microorganisms that live in every human body. Problems arise when yeast becomes unbalanced. Many factors can contribute to this including: medications, diet, genetics, age, hydration, and more. Finding the solution is individual, but the suggestions below may support you on your path to wellness.

. . . .

Tip: Drugs that can wipe out intestinal flora or encourage overgrowth of yeast include steroids and estrogen, either in the form of birth control pills or hormone replacement therapy.

Andrew Weil, MD

. . . .

Our Approach:

Apply: *Melrose* and *Oregano* to the bottoms of the feet.

Oregano is an excellent oil for children, too. Always dilute for kids of course. If you can keep your kids out of the current trend of over-prescribed antibiotics and heavy sugar consumption you will go a long way to avoiding yeast overgrowth in their bodies.

Try: Four drops of **Ocotea** under the tongue before meals, 1 drop of **Clove** on the tip of the tongue to reduce sugar cravings. Try **Alkalime** and **Life 5** probiotic capsules to help create an environment unfavorable for yeast. Try **Essentialzyme** capsules with every meal.

Diffuse: *Peppermint* to clear the mind and reduce cravings.

Mom & Baby note: Thrush usually develops suddenly, but it may become chronic, persisting over a long period of time. A common sign of thrush is the presence of creamy white, slightly raised lesions in your mouth— usually on your tongue or inner cheeks.

Eat an alkaline diet. Alkaline foods include: fresh fruits and vegetables, sea salt, and molasses. Adding probiotics to your routine can keep candida at bay.

Follow our easy program in, *Fat Loss that Works!* Our program gives yeast a run for its money. Eating the right foods keep your body balanced which is the key to managing naturally occurring yeast.

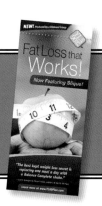

Dear Carrie & Elena,

About a year and a half ago I began getting horrible yeast infections each month right after ovulation right through my menstrual cycle. They were definitely hormonally related because they would go away as soon as my period was over.

But the discomfort was getting more unbearable and each month I could not wait the 2 weeks until it went away. In desperation, I even used OTC yeast infection creams. I began using Progessence Plus about 8 mos. ago for other reasons...but guess what??!!! The yeast infections stopped. I have not had one at all since starting the Progessence Plus...yeah!!!

—Natalie A., NJ

Did You Know?

Candida albicans is a yeast that occurs naturally in the body. The body's natural defenses normally keep yeast in check but if there is an imbalance, yeast can grow out of control. Candida thrives in warm, moist places such as the mouth, vagina, or between folds of the skin.

Cleaning the skin with **Thieves Bar Soap** can keep candida off the skin. Using a topical soap as well as a nutritional supplement and essential oil program can help to balance your body both inside and out.

According to the University of Maryland, about 75 percent of women will get a vaginal yeast infection during their lifetime.

| **Suggested Reading** | *Complete Candida Yeast Guidebook, Revised 2nd Edition: Everything You Need to Know About Prevention, Treatment & Diet* by Jeanne Marie Martin and Zoltan P. Rona M.D. (Paperback, Oct. 12, 2000) | *What to Do When Antibiotics Don't Work! How to Stay Healthy and Alive When Infections Strike* by Dirk Van Gils (Paperback, July 3, 2002) |

Cholesterol

If we are all different then it stands to reason that we should all have different cholesterol levels; however, standard practice today gives everyone the same number. In addition, cholesterol at the right level can play a positive role in the body. Keeping your cholesterol at a healthy level can be supported with oils and nutrition.

·······

Tip: The Harvard Medical School suggests that consuming ½ tsp. of **Cinnamon Bark** a day could reduce cholesterol by 12 to 30 percent. (3 capsules per day.) .

·······

Our Approach:

Apply: One to two drops of **Aroma Life** over the heart and on the bottoms of the feet.

Try: Two ounces of **NingXia Red** with 1 capsule of **Longevity** in the morning and **Essentialzyme** capsules with each meal.

Diffuse: *Lavender* to promote a full nights sleep so that the body can regulate its own cholesterol.

Did you know?

The link between lemongrass and cholesterol was investigated by researchers from the Department of Nutritional Sciences, University of Wisconsin. They published their findings in the medical journal *Lipids* in 1989.

Cholesterol was lowered from 310 to 294 on average--other people in the study experienced a significant decrease in blood fats. The latter group, characterized as responders, experienced a 25-point drop in cholesterol after one month, and this positive trend continued over the course of the short study.

After three months, cholesterol levels among the responders had decreased by a significant 38 points. Once the responders stopped taking lemongrass, their cholesterol returned to previous levels. — CBS News

Essential oils are incredible multi-taskers. Taking an oil for one issue often improves another. We recommend using our fat burning oils to lose weight and reduce your cholesterol.

Try our easy program in the YL90 Plan brochure, *Fat Loss that Works!* Our program gives you a fat burning guide for foods, oils, and supplements.

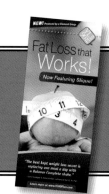

Dear Carrie & Elena,

My husband was diagnosed with high cholesterol and told to go on Statin drugs. Instead I am giving him lemongrass in a capsule everyday and he is feeling more energetic and healthier after only a few days. We are getting his blood work redone in a in a month to see results but we are very optimistic!

—Vicky M., NJ

"I drive way too fast to worry about cholesterol."

—Steven Wright—

| **Suggested Reading** | *Aromatherapy for Health Professionals* by Len Price Cert Ed MIT(Trichology) FISPA FIAM and Shirley Price Cert Ed FISPA MIFA FIAM (Dec 5, 2006) | *The New 8-Week Cholesterol Cure: The Ultimate Program for Preventing Heart Disease* by Robert Kowalski (Dec 24, 2002) | *Reversing Heart Disease: A Vital New Program to Help Prevent, Treat, and Eliminate Cardiac Problems Without Surgery* by Julian M. Whitaker (Mar 1, 2002) |

Cleaning

Essential Oils have been used for cleaning for centuries. Their anti-pathogenic properties keep your home, vehicle, and workplace clean and smelling fresh.

. . . .

Tip: *Melaleuca Alternifolia* and *Grapefruit* are great oils to add to your Thieves cleaning solution or a bucket of soapy water. You can also add these germ killers to sponges, dish water, and the clothes dryer.

. . . .

Our Approach:

Apply: diluted *Thieves Cleaner* to any surface. Always spot test before you proceed. For mold or for tough stains use a 50/50 dilution with water. For glass cleaning add a cup of vinegar and one capful of *Thieves Cleaner* to a 32 oz. spray bottle and fill with water. Different dilutions for different jobs can be found on the bottle. We love the *Thieves Spray* and *Hand Purifier*.

Diffuse: daily. Nothing works better to kill airborne germs and odors than essential oils. Our favorites are: *Thieves*, *Lemon*, *Grapefruit*, *Purification*, and *Citrus Fresh*.

Did you know?

Cleaning with different cleaners can pose a great risk to your health. Cleaning chemicals can linger in the air up to two weeks and when combined with other cleaners can cause a toxic cloud in your home. Residues from cleaners also leave behind dangerous toxins for your children, pets, friends and family to inhale. Synthetic air fresheners can be just as toxic as the odors they attempt to mask.

Thieves cleaner is safe to use, can be used on most surfaces, and will not leave a toxic residue behind in the air or on surfaces.

Greening your home with natural cleaning products is a great way to start improving your health! In our YL90 Plan brochure, *Green Cleaning Solutions*, you will find recipes for cleaning every room in your home.

You will also find ideas on how to green your body with all-natural, essential-oil based personal care products.

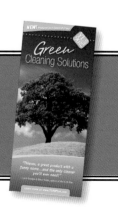

Dear Carrie & Elena,

Thieves is the best cleaner I have ever used. My mother-in-law was a smoker and some things in the house were so stained with nicotine that nothing would clean them. Nothing except Thieves! I had given up on cleaning certain items and once I tried a little swipe of Thieves (without any elbow grease!) the stains vanished!

We are Civil War re-enactors and shoot black powder guns. Thieves is the BEST cleaner for black powder as well! It is not offensive to the nose and safe to use. (It also provides a little oil for the weapon which is necessary for safe operation and maintenance).

I only use Thieves and water to clean everything in my house. This includes my pet sugar glider's cage. He loves when I clean his cage every morning and comes out to play with the sponge and the Thieves. I let him because it is safe for animals. Thieves smells nicely and is pet friendly, too. The breeder had recommended bleach as the only cleaner to use, which is not the safest (for my little guy or anyone else for that matter!) It is so convenient to only use one bottle to do all my cleaning!

—Randy A., NJ,

Shopping List

SINGLES:
Grapefruit
Lemon
Melaleuca Alternifolia
Sacred Frankincense

OIL BLENDS:
Citrus Fresh
Purification
Thieves

HOME CARE:
Thieves Spray
Thieves Cleaner
Thieves Hand Purifier

"Cleaning your house while your children are still growing is like shoveling the sidewalk while it is still snowing!"

—Phyllis Diller—

Suggested Reading

Gorgeously Green: 8 Simple Steps to an Earth-Friendly Life by Sophie Uliano and Julia Roberts (Apr 8, 2008)

'Green This! Greening Your Cleaning' by Deirdre Imus, (Paperback, April 10, 2007)

Nature's Mold Rx, the Non-Toxic Solution to Toxic Mold by Edward R Close, PhD, PE, and Jacquleyn Close, et al. (Paperback, Aug. 31, 2007)

Colds

Common to all of us, colds contribute to more lost work and school days than any other illnesses. Typically lasting 21 days, and caused by viruses, a cold can linger, depressing the spirits as well as the body.

· · · · · · ·

Tip: The key to kicking a cold with essential oils is to start using oils when the first symptom strikes and then repeating often. Frequent use of oils in rotation will make all the difference; aim for every 20 minutes if you can.

· · · · · · ·

Our Approach:

Apply: *Thieves*, *Immupower*, and *Purification* to the feet in rotating order. Apply *RC* and *Raven* to the chest and back. Wipe off household surfaces, including telephones, light switches, and doorknobs, with diluted *Thieves Cleaner*.

Try: Two ounces of **NingXia Red** with an **Inner Defense** capsule (during the day), and a **Life 5** capsule (at night, before bed).

Diffuse: *Thieves* or *Purification* on-and-off all day in the room where you are resting. A cup of boiling water with a few drops of an essential oil can make a great diffuser in a small space or in your workplace.

Did you know?

This "towel" technique has worked for centuries: add boiling water to a bowl and add a few drops of **Eucalyptus Radiata, RC or Raven**. Place a towel over the head to create a steam tent, close your eyes to avoid eye irritation and slowly inhale the aroma for 5 to 10 minutes. Repeat 2-3 times a day until symptoms abate. Adding **Thyme**, **Rosemary**, **Lemon**, or **Thieves** can help loosen mucus and heal the throat, nasal passages and bronchial tubes.

Drink plenty of water when sick. This will help to flush out the cold faster. Try to avoid simple sugars.

Cleaning your home in a "green" way is the best way to avoid colds. Cold bugs are adaptogens, so as our synthetic chemicals kill them, they regroup and become stronger. Essential oils are also adaptogens, so as the pathogens in nature change so do the essential oils that kill them. Your best defense is a good offense.

Learn how to keep a clean green home and body with the YL90 Plan brochure, *Green Cleaning Solutions*.

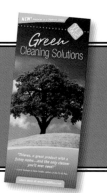

Dear Carrie & Elena,

Last year I had the flu. I started coming down with symptoms on a Tuesday. I started using Thieves on the bottom of my feet and spraying it in my throat in the afternoon.

On Wednesday, I developed a fever so I started diffusing Thieves and Lemon oil; I also applied them topically to my feet every half hour and started to feel a little better. I continued this on Thursday (because I still had a fever) and by Friday was feeling pretty good. The fever was gone and so were most of my symptoms.

By Saturday it was like I never had the flu at all. Most people would have been sick for at least 1-2 weeks with what I had. I know, because I have had this before, and was sick for that long.

—Sean A., NJ

. . . . .

Shopping List

SINGLES:

Eucalyptus Radiata
Lemon
Rosemary
Thyme

OIL BLENDS:

Immupower
Purification
Raven
RC
Thieves

SUPPLEMENTS:

Inner Defense
Life 5
NingXia Red

HOME CARE:

Thieves Cleaner

"A family is a unit composed not only of children but of men, women, an occasional animal, and the common cold."

-Ogden Nash

Suggested Reading

What to Do When Antibiotics Don't Work! How to Stay Healthy and Alive When Infections Strike by Dirk Van Gils (Paperback, July 3, 2002)

Natural Home Health Care Using Essential Oils by Daniel Pénoël, M.D. (Paperback, Aug. 1998)

Congestion

Congestion can be a blocking of the nasal passages due to an inflammation of the membranes lining the nose or from swollen blood vessels of the chest as mucous accumulates.

• • • • • • •

Tip: Apply both *Breathe Again Roll-on* and *Tranquil Roll-on* to the sinuses on either side of the nose. Combined you get the power of a decongestant and an anti-histamine without any of the side effects that a drug would give.

• • • • • • •

Our Approach:

Apply: Warm compresses with **RC, Frankincense**, or **Lavender** over the chest and back. Follow this with **Hyssop**, **Dorado Azul**, or **Raven**. Cover with a warm towel or blanket to keep the body warm.

Try: One to two ounces of **NingXia Red** with an **Inner Defense** capsule (during the day), and a **Life 5** capsule (at night, before bed).

Diffuse: *RC* or *Peppermint* on and off all day in the room where you are resting. A cup of boiling water with a few drops of an essential oil at work can make a great diffuser in a small space.

Did you know?

There are many ways to clear a stuffy nose. Forget Sudafed. An easier, quicker, and cheaper way to relieve sinus pressure is by alternately thrusting your tongue against the roof of your mouth, then pressing between your eyebrows with one finger. This causes the vomer bone, which runs through the nasal passages to the mouth, to rock back and forth, says Lisa DeStefano, D.O., an assistant professor at the Michigan State University College of Osteopathic Medicine. The motion loosens congestion; after 20 seconds, you'll feel your sinuses start to drain.

Congestion relief suggestions in the YL90 Plan brochure, *Allergies, Asthma, & Eczema* can help to relieve your symptoms.

Avoid eating foods made from white flour, white sugar (including soda), chocolate, drinks with caffeine, & dairy products because they provide food for your virus but little nutrition for you. Drink plenty of water and other fluids, both cold & hot (tea, broth, unsweetened juices) especially if the air in your environment is dry.

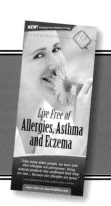

SINGLES:

Dorado Azul
Frankincense
Lavender
Peppermint

OIL BLENDS:

Breathe Again Roll-on
Raven
RC
Tranquil Roll-on

SUPPLEMENTS:

Inner Defense
NingXia Red
Life 5

Dear Carrie & Elena,

When my kids (I have 7, ages 2 to 20) or my husband and I have upper respiratory or nasal congestion or even a cough I put a drop of peppermint oil on a teaspoon with a little honey, agave syrup, or even maple syrup if I have it, on top. It tastes like a peppermint candy and you can breathe clearly right away.

—Ellis O., VA

"*Both of these botanicals [Eucalyptus and Sage] act as an excellent remedy for coughs, chest congestion, and sinus infections. I recommend inhaling the steam made from placing eucalyptus and sage in boiling water at least 2 times a day.*"

—Dr. Andrew Weil—

Suggested Reading   *Most Effective Natural Cures on Earth: The Surprising Unbiased Truth about What Treatments Work and Why* by Jonny Bowden (Jan 1, 2008)

The Essential Oils Handbook: All the Oils You Will Ever Need for Health, Vitality and Well-Being by Jennie Harding (Jun 3, 2008)

Constipation

Constipation refers to bowel movements that are infrequent or hard to pass.

. . . .

Tip: Did you know that as we age we lose our ability to feel thirsty? Getting into a routine where you drink water regularly throughout the day, may help alleviate constipation.

. . . .

Our Approach:

Apply: Warm compresses with a drop of **Di-GIze**, **Peppermint**, or **Ginger** over the abdomen. Use the same oil on the shins and gently massage up and down for 10 minutes to stimulate the digestion. Use a carrier oil like **V6 Mixing Oil** to make the essential oils easier to massage into the skin.

Try: Two oz. of **NingXia Red** & 3-4 drops of **Di-Gize** in a capsule (during the day), and **Comfortone** capsules and a **Life 5** capsule (at night, before bed). Drink plenty of water and avoid binding foods like white flour products, sugar, and chocolate.

Add **Tangerine** to water and drink often throughout the day. Eat plenty of fruits and vegetables. Replace one meal each day with a **Balance Complete** shake.

Did you know?

Constipation is not only caused by many factors, it can lead to other more serious ailments. Do not be afraid to talk to your doctor about irregularity. Bowel movements should occur at least once a day and all bowel movements should be passed without strain.

If you find you develop hemorrhoids, take a few drops of **Melrose** diluted with **V6 Mixing Oil** and gentle apply to the affected area to reduce pain and swelling.

The "clean eating" program found in the YL90 Plan brochure, *Fat Loss that Works*, can not only help you maintain your health and a healthy weight, it can also help you release toxins from your body (which may not be occurring properly if you are suffering from constipation).

Menu suggestions, helpful links, a list of detoxifying foods, and the oils and supplements you need to be regular again are mapped out in this brochure.

Dear Carrie & Elena,

Constipation is a big deal in our family. We take NingXia Red and enzymes to help with proper digestion and we apply Di-Gize and Tangerine to our bellies and our shins to help move things along! We are never without Di-Gize and Tangerine when we're away!

—Dave G., OH

An elderly lady went to her doctor to see what could be done about her constipation.

"It's terrible," she said, "I haven't moved my bowels in a week."

"I see. Have you done anything about it?" asked the doctor.

"Naturally," she replied, "I sit in the bathroom for a half-hour in the morning and again at night."

"No," the doctor said, "I mean do you take anything?"

"Naturally," she answered, "I take a book."

Suggested Reading   *The Essential Oils Handbook: All the Oils You Will Ever Need for Health, Vitality and Well-Being* by Jennie Harding (Jun 3, 2008)   *Better Health Through Natural Healing: How to Get Well Without Drugs or Surgery* by Ross Trattler and Adrian Jones (Aug 2004)

Cough

We all know how painful and disruptive a cough can be; some are dry, others wet, some can be productive, others will cause a spam that seems to never end. You may need to try 2 or 3 oils to find the right combination for your cough.

. . . .

Tip: Comparing and reviewing 25 studies on over-the-counter cough medicine, a recent research review published in The Cochrane Library determined that there's no good evidence for or against the effectiveness of formulas such as Robitussin and Mucinex.

. . . .

Our Approach:

Apply: Warm compresses with *RC*, *Eucalyptus Globulus*, *Eucalyptus Blue*, *Frankincense*, or *Lavender* over the chest and back. Follow this with *Hyssop*, *Dorado Azul*, or *Raven*. Apply one drop *Peppermint* on top to drive in the other oils. Cover with a warm towel or blanket to keep the body warm.

Try: One ounce of *NingXia Red* & an *Inner Defense* capsule (during the day), and a *Life 5* capsule (at night before bed). One drop of *Lemon* oil on a spoon with honey or agave syrup on top can make a quick throat soother and tastes like a lemon drop candy.

Diffuse: *RC* or *Peppermint* on and off all day in the room where you are resting. A cup of boiling water with a few drops of an essential oil at work can make a great diffuser in a small space.

Did you know?

I think most will agree, nighttime can be the worst enemy of the person with a cough. Getting to sleep and staying asleep can be the difference between getting better and staying sick. Be sure to take *ImmuPro* capsules at least ½ hour before bed to relax the body and support the immune system in addition to using your oils for cough and sleep. We like *Lavender* on the feet and *RC* on the chest and back. Need something stronger? Apply *RutaVaLa Roll-on* and *Stress Away Roll-on* to the spine.

The YL90 Plan brochure, *Cold-n-Flu Fighters,* is your complete guide to dealing with all your cold symptoms including the worst of coughs.

If you can stop the beginning symptoms like a runny nose or post nasal drip, you may be able to avoid a cough from developing.

If you tend to start a cold with a cough, learn how to keep your lungs strong all year long.

Dear Carrie & Elena,

What I have found to alleviate bronchial infections is alternating between Thieves, RC and Eucalyptus in a diffuser and a couple of drops on my chest. It has helped subside my chronic coughing to subside making it possible to get some rest. During the fall I always have it diffusing in my son's room to help him. I notice that when I do that for him, his coughing subsides also.

—Leila R., NJ

"When at a loss how to go on, in speaking, cough"

—Greek proverb—

| **Suggested Reading** | Natural Home Remedies: Safe and Effective Treatments for Common Ailments by Karen Sullivan (Hardcover, 1997) | Aromatherapy for the Healthy Child: More Than 300 Natural, Nontoxic, and Fragrant Essential Oil Blends by Valerie Ann Worwood (Paperback, Mar. 9, 2000) |

Cuts, Scrapes, & Bruises

Whether a cut, scrape, or bruise the first line of attack must be to prevent infection and the second to heal the skin quickly and without scarring.

• • • • • • •

Tip: Using a "triple antibiotic" cream for minor cuts is like using a sledgehammer to crack a walnut. A simpler alternative, **Melaleuca Alternifolia**, can be applied straight to the skin and is a natural antiseptic, antibacterial, and germicide, fungicide.

— *Journal of Hospital Infection*

• • • • • • •

Our Approach:

Apply: A clean warm cloth to the hurt area to remove any debris. Spritz with **Lavaderm Spray** and apply **Melrose** topically and cover if necessary. Once the wound is closed, apply **Lavender**, **Frankincense**, and **Helichrysum** to prevent scaring.

Try: A **Super B** tablet & **True Source** vitamins to promote healing of the skin.

Diffuse: *Peace & Calming* if you have trouble sleeping or if shaken from the trauma.

Did you know?

The injury required to produce a bruise varies with age. While it may take quite a bit of force to cause a bruise in a young child, even minor bumps and scrapes may cause extensive bruising or ecchymosis in an elderly person. Blood vessels become more fragile as we age, and bruising may even occur without prior injury in the elderly.

The amount of bruising may also be affected by medications. Do your homework and be sure to understand how your medications may affect you.

Kids get into a lot of "scrapes." The information found in the YL90 Plan, *Kids, Teens, & Tots* is good for children and adults alike. Getting the oils on the body as soon as possible is key. Be sure to carry your "first aid" oils with you so that you always have what you need.

Adhesive strips will not stick to the skin once essential oils are applied. Apply a gauze pad or allow the skin to dry before covering with an adhesive strip.

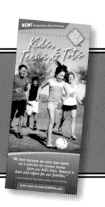

Dear Carrie & Elena,

When my son was a small toddler, he was standing by a door and someone opened it not knowing that he was there. He got hit in the forehead and I could see a big bruise forming. I immediately applied lavender to the bruise and I could actually see the blue color slowly fading in front of my eyes. I put him down for his nap and after it had no trace of a bruise.

A few days later, my son ran into a door frame and bruised his forehead again on the same spot. I had loaned the lavender oil to my sister and didn't have it to apply on my son's forehead. Well, he ended up getting a big bruise which turned blue and then yellow and stayed discolored for a couple of weeks. What a contrast to our experience when we did have the lavender oil.

—Tim P., NJ

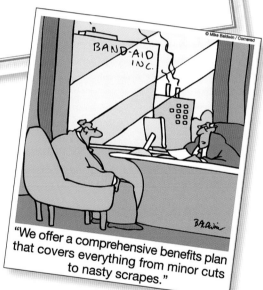

© Mike Baldwin / Cornered

"We offer a comprehensive benefits plan that covers everything from minor cuts to nasty scrapes."

Suggested Reading

Aromatherapy for the Healthy Child: More Than 300 Natural, Nontoxic, and Fragrant Essential Oil Blends by Valerie Ann Worwood (Paperback, Mar. 9, 2000)

Aroma: The International Magazine for Essential Oils. Nr. 1/ Winter 2000: Lavender by Terra Linda Scent and Image Inc. (Hardcover, 2000)

The Complete Illustrated Guide to Natural Home Remedies by C. Norman Shealey Karen Sullivan (2010)

Dental Health

Dental health reaches beyond just your teeth and gums. Maintain the health of your teeth, gums, tongue and even your throat to insure good dental and overall health.

. . . .

Tip: Try all 4 Young Living toothpastes to find the right one for you. Do not assume if someone in your family does not care for the taste of one, they will not like the others. Add one to each of your orders until you find your favorite.

. . . .

Our Approach:

Apply: *Thieves* and *Sacred Frankincense* to gums 1-4 times a month. *Thieves* is also great for mild toothaches and infections. Brush daily with *Thieves toothpaste* (*Dentarome*, *Dentarome Plus*, *Dentarome Ultra*, or *Kidscents Toothpaste*). Rinse with *Thieves Mouthwash*.

Try: *Alkalime* daily to maintain good pH balance in the body and support dental health. Substitute one meal a day with a *Balance Complete* shake. Before every meal take *Essentialzyme* capsules for better digestion.

Diffuse: *Peace & Calming* before your visit to the dentist to calm any nervous tension you may be feeling.

Did you know?

Here's some great information from Holistic Dental Association: Preventing periodontal disease (a disease of the gums and bone that support the teeth) with brushing and flossing can help prevent heart disease. According to the American Academy of Periodontology, people with periodontal (gum) disease are almost twice as likely to have coronary artery disease (also called heart disease). One study found that the presence of common problems in the mouth, including gum disease (gingivitis), cavities, and missing teeth, were as good at predicting heart disease as cholesterol levels.

Clean eating is one way to improve your dental health. Avoiding sticky and processed foods will lower the acidity in your body and keep teeth strong. Replace these foods with fat burning foods that also protect your teeth and you get a double bonus!

Try our easy program in the YL90 Plan brochure, *Fat Loss that Works!* Our program provides you with great meal suggestions and other clean eating resources.

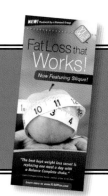

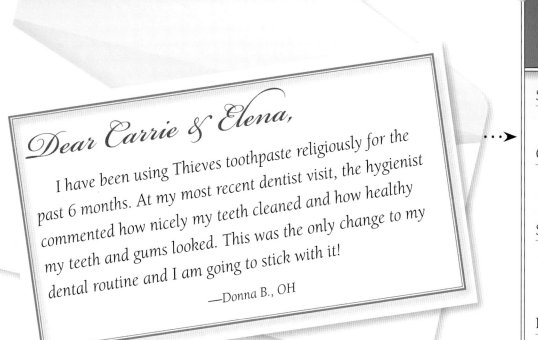

Dear *Carrie & Elena,*

I have been using Thieves toothpaste religiously for the past 6 months. At my most recent dentist visit, the hygienist commented how nicely my teeth cleaned and how healthy my teeth and gums looked. This was the only change to my dental routine and I am going to stick with it!

—Donna B., OH

"You don't have to brush your teeth – just the ones you want to keep."

—Author Unknown—

Suggested Reading

Reversing Gum Disease Naturally: A Holistic Home Care Program by Sandra Senzon, RDH (Paperback, April 25, 2003)

The Aromatherapy Encyclopedia: A Concise Guide to over 385 Plant Oils by Carol Schiller, David Schiller and Jeffrey Schiller (Jun 15, 2008)

Healing Oils Of The Bible by David Stewart (Paperback, Apr. 25, 2004)

Depression

Depression effects one out of every three Americans and unfortunately is rising every year. Medications may have a temporary effect but are also associated with many unpleasant side effects.

. . . .

Tip: Eliminating sugars and refined food from your diet can help end feelings of lethargy and despair. Although high-carbohydrate foods like biscuits and cakes can be comforting initially, they play havoc with your blood sugar levels and can leave you feeling tired and sad soon after eating them.

. . . .

Our Approach:

Apply: *Harmony*, *Joy*, *White Angelica*, *and Valor* 2-3 times a day over the heart, on the wrists, and on the feet.

Try: Four ounces of **NingXia Red**; and 3 **OmegaGize** capsules, 3 times a day. Take **Essentialzyme** capsules with every meal, **Sleepessence** capsules, and a **Super B** tablet at night to prevent middle-of-the-night waking.

Diffuse: **Citrus Fresh** to uplift the spirits, or **Peace & Calmng** to relax.

Did you know?

Everyday tasks can seem overwhelming to someone with depression. Mixing the 4 oils (listed under "Apply") and putting them in an empty roll-on bottle can make using the oils easier. Making a roll-on for your loved one can be one of the best gifts you can give them.

Almost all of the vitamins in the B group play an active role in tackling depression. Vitamin B1 (thiamine) and B2 (riboflavin) deficiencies have been linked to depression; while vitamin B3 (niacinamide) has been used to treat depression because it can increase serotonin levels. Seratonin is a neurotransmitter that helps relay messages from one side of the brain to the other. Without it, it can be hard to balance our mood. Vitamin B6 (pyridoxine) is also needed for the conversion of the amino acid tryptophan to serotonin (Psych Res 1980 3(2) 141-150). Taking a **Super B** tablet 1-2 times a day is a great way to get the B vitamins you need.

The YL90 Plan brochure, *End the Blues,* is written for those with any degree of anxiety or depression. Although this is a 90-day plan, it can be used on a ongoing basis until you feel like your emotions have leveled.

Each person's chemistry is different. The amount of time you will need to get your body balanced can vary. Use the products for at least 90 days and then slowly decrease the amount of product you are using to find the level that you need to keep your body balanced.

Dear Carrie & Elena,

In 2005 I was on anti-depressant and anti-anxiety medication. They did their job of pulling me out of a deep funk and allowed me to function. However, after my mood was stabilized, I started to feel numb. I could not feel anything. Situations that should have made me sad didn't and situations that should have made me joyful didn't either. I felt like the typical teenager and "whatever" was my response to just about everything.

I began to drink 1 ounce of NingXia Red daily. I started using Valor on my wrists, Joy over my heart, Harmony over my solar plexus and White Angelica on the crown of my head. I used one drop of each oil a few times a day and was able to quit my meds. I didn't feel too well the first week but I knew I was doing the right thing and that eventually I would start to feel better. By week two, the old, animated me was re-emerging and I began to lose that numb, zombie like feeling. Fast forward 6 years. I feel so much better and don't even feel the need to use the program every day.

—Lorinda Walker, Essential Wellness and Massage Therapy, NJ

"Too often we underestimate the power of a touch, a smile, a kind word, a listening ear, an honest compliment, or the smallest act of caring, all of which have the potential to turn a life around."

—Leo Buscaglia—

Suggested Reading

Releasing Emotional Patterns with Essential Oils by Carolyn L. Mein (Paperback, Sept. 1, 1998)

Healing Oils, Healing Hands 2nd Edition by Linda L Smith (Paperback, June 30, 2008)

Aromatherapy for Healing the Spirit: Restoring Emotional and Mental Balance with Essential Oils by Gabriel Mojay (Jan 1, 2000)

Diabetes

Diabetes is a disease in which your blood glucose, (also called blood sugar), levels are too high. Glucose comes from the foods we eat. Insulin is a hormone that helps the glucose get into your cells to give them energy. With Type 1 diabetes, your body does not make insulin. With Type 2 diabetes, the more common type, the body does not use insulin well, causing the glucose to stay in the blood instead of going into cells where it is needed.

Our Approach:

Apply: *Dill* and *Cypress*, to the bottoms of the feet, 2 times daily.

Try: Four drops of *Ocotea* or *Cinnamon Bark* under the tongue before meals. For sugar cravings, try 1 drop of *Clove* on the tip of the tongue. To promote healthy eating substitute one meal a day with a *Balance Complete* shake and take *Essentialzyme* capsules before each meal to help improve digestion and nutrient absorption

Diffuse: *Peppermint* to clear the mind and reduce cravings.

Did you know?

The CDC (Center for Disease Control) estimates that as many as 1 in 3 U.S. adults could have diabetes by 2050 if current trends continue. Type 2 diabetes, in which the body gradually loses its ability to use insulin properly, accounts for 90% to 95% of cases.

"Using natural product screening, chemists have discovered the only blockbuster diabetes drug: cinnamon. Cinnamon is positioned to save modern society from the type 2 diabetes epidemic." Wellbeing Journal May/June 2011. We find *Ocotea*, in the cinnamon family, to be the best of the cinnamon oils on the market today.

Clinical trials have shown that losing just 5 to 7 percent of body weight – that's 10 to 14 pounds for a 200-pound person – and getting at least 150 minutes of moderate physical activity each week reduces the risk of type 2 diabetes by nearly 60 percent in those at high risk for developing the disease. —Centers for Disease Control

Try our easy program in the YL90 Plan brochure, *Fat Loss that Works!* Our program gives you a fat burning guide for foods, oils, and supplements.

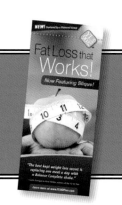

SINGLES:

Cassia
Cinnamon Bark
Clove
Cypress
Dill
Ocotea
Peppermint

SUPPLEMENTS:

Balance Complete
Essentialzyme
Mineral Essence

Dear Carrie & Elena,

I was diagnosed as "pre-diabetic" in December 2009. After seeing a nutritionist and cutting out all white flour and sugar and increasing my exercise I was discouraged to discover that my numbers weren't changing, despite all the lifestyle changes. I finally agreed to try some "natural stuff" my wife recommended in March but only one capsule a day in the morning with three drops in it.

I tested my blood before and after the capsule. The blood sugar consistently went down at least 10 points within 10 minutes of taking 3 drops of Ocotea.

I also take 2 OmegaGize capsules and about 2 ounces of Ningxia Red in addition to the 3 drops of Ocotea essential oil. In June, (3 months later) I went for my blood work and the doctor said my numbers were so good I was no longer considered diabetic. Needless to say, I'm ecstatic! I'm convinced it was the diet as well as the Ocotea that made the difference.

—John G., NJ

Tip: Carry *Ocotea*, **Cassia**, or **Cinnamon Bark** (all in the cinnamon family) with you. Take one drop of one of these oils under the tongue before eating anything to help regulate blood sugar.

. . . .

Everything is a miracle. It is a miracle that one does not dissolve like a lump of sugar.

—Pablo Picasso—

Suggested Reading

There Is a Cure for Diabetes: The Tree of Life 21-Day+ Program by Gabriel Cousens (Paperback, Jan. 8, 2008)

The Johns Hopkins Guide to Diabetes: For Today and Tomorrow (A Johns Hopkins Press Health Book) by Christopher D. Saudek, Richard R. Rubin and Cynthia S. Shump (Jun 12, 1997)

Reversing Diabetes by Julian M. Whitaker (Nov 1, 2009)

Diarrhea

No matter the cause, the biggest threat to the body from diarrhea is dehydration. Keeping liquids in the body is key to the healing process. Oils can help play a key roll in keeping the body from dehydrating.

• • • • • • •

Tip: Addressing your diet and stress levels rather than popping pills is often the safer and more effective route. Go the Natural Route! Stomach acid decreases with age and it's important to maintain what you do have. Acid-blocking drugs like Pepcid & Zantac are incredibly overprescribed (Mullin).

• • • • • • •

Our Approach:

Apply: Two drops of **Di-Gize** to the abdomen either neat or diluted. Apply often at first and then consistently every (2-4 hours) for at least 24 hours after the diarrhea has subsided.

Try: A drop of **Peppermint** or **Ginger** in water until diarrhea has subsided. Then, take 1 shot of **NingXia Red** with a dropper full of **Mineral Essence** every hour to replace electrolytes. Drink water in small doses to replace what has been lost.

Diffuse: **Peppermint** to settle the stomach.

Did you know?

Manage Stress—That feeling of butterflies in your stomach has a physiological basis. "There's a lot of cross talk between the brain and the gut," explains James Mullin, Ph.D., a clinical neuropsychologist. Your GI tract has its own nervous system, which is why stress can cause digestive problems such as diarrhea, heartburn, and irritable bowel syndrome (IBS). Learn to manage stress -- and reduce GI problems —by exploring massage, art therapy, breathing exercises, and other relaxation techniques.

The YL90 Plan brochure, *Cold-N-Flu Fighters*, has a complete guide to symptom relief for all your needs.

This easy-to-follow symptom relief guide will provide all the direction you need to use your products effectively. Remember to keep these commonly needed products on hand so that you have them when a bug strikes!

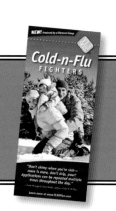

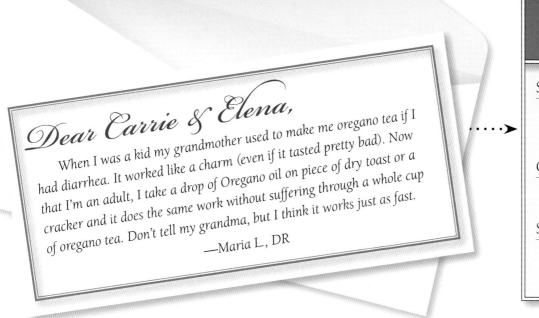

Dear Carrie & Elena,

When I was a kid my grandmother used to make me oregano tea if I had diarrhea. It worked like a charm (even if it tasted pretty bad). Now that I'm an adult, I take a drop of Oregano oil on piece of dry toast or a cracker and it does the same work without suffering through a whole cup of oregano tea. Don't tell my grandma, but I think it works just as fast.

—Maria L., DR

Join the Culture Club—"Your digestive tract is a delicate ecosystem of both good and bad bacteria," says David Rakel, MD. When you eat a lot of processed food or take antibiotics, you can wipe out these "friendly" bacteria. This allows the bad guys to take over, leading to IBS, diarrhea, and other problems. Maintain a healthy balance of bacteria by eating a daily cup of yogurt labeled "contains active cultures," if you have digestive problems, Mullin recommends, and taking a probiotic supplement that includes good bacteria.

> *"It is still just unbelievable to us that diarrhea is one of the leading causes of child deaths in the world."*
>
> —Melinda Gates—

Suggested Reading

The Aromatherapy Encyclopedia: A Concise Guide to over 385 Plant Oils by Carol Schiller, David Schiller and Jeffrey Schiller (Jun 15, 2008)

The Maker's Diet: The 40-day health experience that will change your life forever by Jordan Rubin (Paperback, Mar 31, 2005)

Digestion

Digestive issues run the gamut from an upset stomach after overeating or eating the wrong foods to a serious chronic disorder such as Crohn's Disease or Irritable Bowel Syndrome and chronic constipation.

· · · · · · ·

Tip: Dr. Andrew Weil says, "Plant-derived digestive enzymes (for example bromelain, derived from pineapples) can help digest specific nutrients." Our favorite enzyme complexes are contained in ***Essentialzyme***.

· · · · · · ·

Our Approach:

Apply: Two drops of ***Di-Gize, Ginger*** or ***Peppermint*** on the abdomen on a daily basis, more often if problems are severe. Roll-on ***Stress Away*** to reduce the stress of a chronic disorder.

Try: ***Essentialzyme*** capsules with meals & a ***Life 5*** capsule at night to promote good digestion and healthy bowel movements. Take a ***Digest & Cleanse*** capsule between meals for extra support.

Diffuse: ***Peace & Calming*** day and night to help reduce stress and lessen the stress on the digestive tract.

Did you know?

Ulcers can be caused by diet, stress, or pathogens. No matter what the cause, bringing the digestive system into proper balance should help to lessen, or even heal, ulcers and other stomach aliments such as reflux and flatulence.

Eating a diet rich in fruits, vegetables, and enzymes helps to promote proper digestion. Try blending fresh foods into smoothies and soups if you find them hard to digest. Adding ***Alkalime*** to alkaline the body will help with issues caused by too much acid. ***Life 5*** probiotics at night will help replenish good bacteria in the gut. ***Essentialzyme*** capsules with meals will help digest foods more completely to ease digestion. ***Stress Away Roll-on*** used daily will help to keep stress from attacking the digestive system. Try any of the above to find the formula that works best for you.

Knowing how to apply, ingest, and diffuse essential oils can help with good digestion.

Follow our guidelines in this "basics" brochure to learn how to use and share your essential oils most effectively.

The YL90 Plan brochure, *Essential Oil Basics*, will get you started and keep you moving forward!

Dear Carrie & Elena,

Whenever I am nauseous or have any kind of stomach upset a drop or two of Di-Gize rubbed on my belly does the trick. Usually, I feel better within five minutes of using Di-Gize this way. If I don't feel better after ten minutes, I drink a glass of water with a drop of Di-Gize in it, take a drop of Ginger on my tongue, or inhale Peppermint and that works quickly. Di-Gize, Ginger, and Peppermint are my go-to oils for all types of gastrointestinal distress.

—Laura P., PR

Shopping List

SINGLES:
Ginger
Peppermint

OIL BLENDS:
Di-Gize
Peace & Calming
Stress Away Roll-on

SUPPLEMENTS:
Alkalime
Essentialzyme
Life 5
NingXia Red

"Do not worry; eat three square meals a day; say your prayers;
be courteous to your creditors; keep your digestion good; exercise;
go slow and easy. Maybe there are other things your special case requires
to make you happy, but my friend, these I reckon will give you a good lift."

—Abraham Lincoln—

Suggested Reading

The Complete Book of Enzyme Therapy: A Complete and Up-to-Date Reference to Effective Remedies by Anthony J. Cichoke (Paperback, Nov 15, 1998)

Clinical Aromatherapy: Essential Oils in Practice, Second Edition by Jane Buckle (Paperback, Jun 11, 2003)

Healing Oils Of The Bible by David Stewart (Paperback, May 12, 2004)

Earaches

Although common in children, earaches can occur at any age. Often caused by inflammation, dehydration, or an over proliferation of pathogens, pain can range from minor to debilitating.

"People think earwax is dirt. It's not dirt. It's a protective coating for our ear canal."

—Rick Friedman, a neurotologist at the House Clinic in Los Angeles.

• • • • • • •

Tip: Apply *PanAway* around the ear to lessen the pain and reduce swelling. Essential oils can help diminish pain safely. **Never put essential oils into the ear!**

• • • • • • •

Our Approach:

Apply: Around the ear (never in) *Palo Santo*, *Melrose*, and *Grapefruit*. Dilute these with *V6 Mixing Oil* if the skin around the ear becomes red or irritated.

Try: Drinking 2 oz. of *NingXia Red* & take an *Inner Defense* capsule during the day and a *Life 5* capsule at night. Drinking water with *Lemon* or *Citrus Fresh* will help to flush out toxins.

Diffuse: *Lavender* for its germ fighting and relaxing qualities.

Did you know?

"In the past 10 years, there has been a recognition that we don't hear just with the ears. We hear with the brain," says Barbara Cone, a professor of speech, language, and hearing sciences at the University of Arizona, in Tucson. The brain's job is not only to receive sound but also to reduce background noise and hone in on the things we most want to hear -- quite often, other people's voices. Human ears are particularly attuned to the frequency range used in conversation. Our large brain and long life span enable us to use our experiences to differentiate an extraordinary variety of sounds.

Whether focusing on symptom relief or working on the root cause, an easy application of oils can do wonders to relieve an earache. Be sure to apply often. Many times people do not get the results they desire because they are not using their oils often enough.

Follow the YL90 Plan brochure, *Kids, Teens, & Tots*, for earaches and don't be afraid to use your oils every 10-20 minutes the first day.

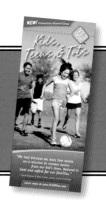

Dear Carrie & Elena,

One night my son came to me in the middle of the night crying that his ear was hurting him very badly. I put Purification on a piece of cotton and put it in his ear. Then I rubbed around his ear with lavender. He went back to sleep and woke up the next morning with no more pain and went to school. (Other times when an earache was more severe, it took several applications every couple of hours. Then the earache was gone in 24 hours.)

—Mary H, WI

An Ear Full - Or Not?

Hazel went to her family physician with her crying baby. The doctor diagnosed right away that the baby had an earache and wrote a prescription for ear drops. In the directions he wrote, 'Put two drops in right ear every four hours', and he abbreviated "right" as an R with a circle around it.

Hazel returned to the doctor after several days and complained that the baby still had an earache, but his bottom was getting really greasy with all those drops of oil.

The doctor was perplexed and looked at the bottle of ear drops and realized immediately what had gone wrong. The Pharmacist had typed the following instructions on the label:

'Put two drops in R ear every four hours.'

Suggested Reading	*Gentle Babies: Essential Oils and Natural Remedies for Pregnancy, Childbirth, Infants and Young Children* (Third Edition) by Debra Raybern (Paperback - 2010)
	Aromatherapy for the Healthy Child: More Than 300 Natural, Nontoxic, and Fragrant Essential Oil Blends by Valerie Ann Worwood (Paperback, Mar. 9, 2000)

Energy

Energy comes from the body's ability to process what we eat and turn it into energy we can use. When we eat the wrong food our body cannot process we can end up being tired and sluggish. This can actually lead to sleepless nights which compound exhaustion. Once run down, we are vulnerable to illness which can weaken us further.

. . . .

Tip: Take your minerals at night. Minerals are great promoters of sleep which can give you more energy during the day.

. . . .

Our Approach:

Apply: A few drops of **En-R-Gee** to the back of the neck. **Peppermint, Rosemary**, and **Basil**, are also great pick-me-ups.

Try: A **Super B** tablet & **True Source** vitamins right before the most tiring part of your day. For energy that is healthy and will last, try **NingXia Red** & **Multigreen** capsules instead of coffee and chocolate.

Diffuse: **Peppermint, Clarity** or **Lemon**, in a room where you are working. This can help keep your energy high and mind alert.

Did you know?

You can get an energy boost by stretching while diffusing oils.

1. Sit with your legs extended straight in front of you, feet parallel with toes pointing up. Press the back of your legs into the floor.

2. Inhale deeply and lift through the upper body. With your spine straight and shoulders back, pull the navel in slightly toward the spine, creating space in the abdomen. Exhale, release, and lean forward, bending from the hip, not the waist.

One key effect of getting a Raindrop treatment is detoxification. No matter what may be off balance in your body, a Raindrop treatment can jump-start your system and give your body a boost of energy.

Following the YL90 Plan for nutritional support between Raindrop treatments in our brochure, (*Who Needs A Raindrop? Everybody!*), can give you the support you need to continue your detox and reach the energy level you desire.

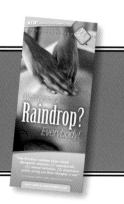

Dear Carrie & Elena,

I have been using essential oils daily for over 3 years and regularly for over 15 years. Oils have helped me with many problems both big and small. I love the blend Clarity. I keep a small diffuser by my desk in the office and I diffuse throughout the day. My colleagues often pass my door and remark, "Tu sens si bon!" (You smell so good.) I find that diffusing helps to keep my energy up and my mind focused.

I also use Geranium as a perfume that lifts my spirits if they are flagging. My students love it too. I frequently use Lavender in class to keep everyone acting as they should and focused on the lesson.

—Guitty R., France

Shopping List

SINGLES:
- Basil
- Lemon
- Peppermint
- Rosemary

OIL BLENDS:
- Clarity
- En-R-Gee

SUPPLEMENTS:
- Multigreens
- NingXia Red
- Super B
- True Source

3. Fold forward only as far as you can (keep your knees bent if that's more comfortable). With each inhalation, lift and lengthen the front torso slightly; if you feel able to go further, release a little more fully into the bend on an exhale. Try not to crunch; maintain length through the spine.

4. Hold for a few breaths, allowing your body to open up. Direct your breath toward the kidneys, breathing deep into the lower back. Then inhale and sit up slowly, lifting your torso away from the thighs until your back is straight. Repeat 2 to 3 times.

The more you lose yourself in something bigger than yourself, the more energy you will have."

—Normal Vincent Peale—

Suggested Reading

Chi-To-Be by Stacey Hall (Paperback, 2011)
Healing Oils, Healing Hands 2nd Edition by Linda L Smith (Paperback, Jun 30, 2008)

Discovery of the Ultimate Superfood: How the Ningxia Wolfberry And 4 Other Foods Help Combat Heart Disease, Cancer, Chronic Fatigue, Depression, Diabetes And More by Gary Young, Marc Schreuder and Ronald, Ph.D. Lawrence (Paperback, July 30, 2005)

Feet, Hands, & Nails

The eyes are the windows to the soul, but the hands, nails, and feet are the measure of age. You can hide your age almost everywhere else, but your hands, nails, and feet will usually give you away. A true indicator of improving health is the appearance of your feet, hands, and nails.

Tip: Essential oils are very effective in fighting warts and fungus. Apply *Melaleuca Alternifolia*, *Thieves*, *Oregano*, or *Lemongrass*, and let air dry.

Our Approach:

Apply: *Peppermint Cedarwood Soap* once a week to wash hands and feet. Moisturize cuticles and nails with **Myrrh** and **Rose Ointment**. Apply **Cypress** to hands and feet to improve circulation. Apply **Animal Scents Ointment** to soften and heals callouses.

Try: Two oz. of *NingXia Red* with *Sulfurzyme* capsules, and *OmegaGize* capsules daily. These supplements can help rejuvenate tired hands and feet and restore a youthful appearance.

Diffuse: *Lavender* or *Frankincense* at night. The calming effects of these oils are very supportive of hand and feet health.

Did you know?

That Methylsulfonylmethane, (MSM, found in **Sulfurzyme**) has long been studied for its effects on nail health? In a double-blind, placebo-controlled, pilot trial, conducted simultaneously, showed that 50% of the subjects on MSM showed increased nail length and nail thickness growth compared to the group on a placebo. —Ronald M. Lawrence, M.D., Ph.D

Summer is a great time to start taking care of your hands and feet. Everyone wants to put their best foot forward--especially in sandals.

Follow the YL90 Plan guide in our brochure, *Enjoy The Great Outdoors*, for tips on how to care for your hands, nails, and feet in the summer and all year long!

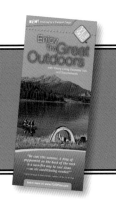

Dear Carrie & Elena,

I had tried and failed to cure a fungal infection in three toenails for over two years with a prescription nail lacquer. I was recommended Animal Scents Ointment and Melaleuca were recommended to me, so I tried them. Within a week or so there was a noticeable improvement and after a month, the nail growth could clearly show the nail growing free from the infection. This is recent, so the nail still has to grow fully, but I am very pleased so far with the result!

—Mark W., NJ

"For days after death, hair and fingernails continue to grow, but phone calls taper off."

—Johnny Carson—

Did you know?

The "side benefit" of taking **Sulfurzyme** is a decrease in inflammation, the root cause of all disease. Following calcium and phosphorus, sulfur is the third most abundant mineral in the body. It is a strong anti-oxidant, detoxifier, & analgesic. Studies have shown its positive effects on cancer, autoimmune diseases, allergies, digestive disorders, pain, diabetes, & stress.

—Dr. Stanley Jacob and Dr. Robert Herschler, *MSM The Definitive Guide*

....

Shopping List

SINGLES:

Cypress
Frankincense
Lavender
Lemongrass
Melaleuca Alternifolia
Myrrh
Oregano

OIL BLENDS:

Thieves

SUPPLEMENTS:

NingXia Red
OmegaGize
Sulfurzyme

PERSONAL CARE:

Animal Scents
Ointment
Rose Ointment
Peppermint
    Cedarwood Soap

Suggested Reading

A Consumer's Dictionary of Cosmetic Ingredients, 7th Edition: by Ruth Winter (Paperback, Oct 20, 2009)

500 Formulas for Aromatherapy by Carol Schiller and David Schiller (Paperback, June 30, 1994)

Making Aromatherapy Creams and Lotions: 101 Natural Formulas to Revitalize & Nourish Your Skin by Donna Maria (Paperback, Jul 15, 2000)

Fever

A fever is an elevation of body temperature. This happens when the body is trying to kill off a pathogen. As a fever increases or is sustained for a prolonged period of time it is important to seek medical attention right away.

· · · · · · ·

Tip: Remember to drink plenty of water and eat lightly when feeling feverish. This gives the body extra support to fight illness and recover quickly.

· · · · · · ·

Our Approach:

Apply: A few drops of *Lavender*, *Peppermint*, and *Lemon*, to the back of the neck and on the bottom of the feet every 10-20 minutes until a fever subsides.

Try: One shot of *NingXia Red* & 1 *Inner Defense* capsule 2-3 times a day.

Diffuse: *Peace & Calming* or *Lavender* to help you sleep and recover.

Did you know?

A fever can be a good indication that an infection may be present. Drugs stop the fever immediately, but also stop the body's "alert system." The application of essential oils fight infections, viruses, and other germs with the fever. These oils include: *Oregano*, *Thyme*, *Mountain Savory*, *Thieves*, *Melrose*, and *Immupower*.

A low fever can actually benefit a sick child. The body is trying to do the right thing. Most bacteria & viruses like to live at body temperature. So if the temperature is raised, "bugs" are killed off. Research shows that parental tendencies to "fever phobia" -- a fear that fever is harmful -- originated after the introduction of anti-fever drugs like Tylenol and Advil.

Nothing will make a parent more nervous than a child with a fever. Though conventional wisdom tells us there is nothing to worry about, no one wants their child to suffer.

Use the easy guide to fever and other symptom relief in our YL90 Plan brochure, *Cold-N-Flu Fighters*. From fever to coughs, this brochure will be your go-to guide for helping your children feel better fast.

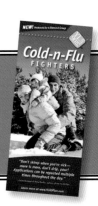

Shopping List

....

SINGLES:

Lavender
Lemon
Mountain Savory
Oregano
Peppermint
Thyme

OIL BLENDS:

Immupower
Melrose
Peace & Calming
Thieves

SUPPLEMENTS:

Inner Defense
NingXia Red

Dear Carrie & Elena,

I am a mom of young children under the age of 5 and a massage therapist. Fevers are common in our house and I try to treat them naturally instead of using over the counter meds. For us, Peppermint works to lower a fever, combined with Lavender, Wintergreen, and Basil. On a baby, I use Lavender, mostly on the feet, with a little Peppermint. I alternate feet and neck, if the fever climbs. After applying, I hold the feet for 5 to 10 min. Oils only on the feet didn't always work for us. In that case, I would apply the oils to the neck and spine, too, in order to bring down a fever. Hope this helps other moms.

—Kerry B., NJ

"There is no such thing as a life of passion any more than a continuous earthquake, or an eternal fever."

—Lord Byron—

| **Suggested Reading** | *The Complete Illustrated Guide to Natural Home Remedies* by C. Norman Shealey Karen Sullivan (2010)

Growing up Green, Kids & Teens by Dierdre Imus (Paperback) | *Gentle Babies: Essential Oils and Natural Remedies for Pregnancy, Childbirth, Infants and Young Children* (Third Edition) by Debra Raybern (Paperback, 2010) |

Focus

In a world constantly pulling us in hundreds of directions, focus is a daily challenge. Calming the nervous system and quieting the mind is key.

. . . .

Tip: The mind works best in 20 minute increments. Give yourself a break, even for a minute or two while you are working on long-term projects. You will be amazed at how much more productive you become. A timer is a great tool.

. . . .

Our Approach:

Apply: *Clarity* to the temples and back of the neck and *Brain Power* to the big toes.

Try: *Core Supplements* and drink **NingXia Red** daily. Feeding your brain with good nutrition will keep your mind focused.

Diffuse: *Peppermint* when you need to concentrate, study, or work for long periods of time.

Did you know?

Some scientists suspect we get better at complex reasoning in our forties and fifties because that's when our brain's white matter peaks, says George Bartzokis, M.D., who studies age-related dementia at UCLA, in terms any brain could understand.

"Think of your brain as the Internet," he says. "Half consists of the computer, or the gray matter. The other half is what we call white matter. It's made up of axons, or wires, which take information away from the neurons, and myelin, which is like the insulation around the wires."

Myelin, helps increase transmission from one cell body to another. Some studies indicate that the facts we've accumulated don't get lost; they simply fall between the cushions like peanuts, and we have to work to dig them out.

Do you have a plan? One can't focus without one. We spend so much of our time worrying and wondering which significantly cuts into our productivity.

Whether using the YL90 Plan for a health or business goal, you will find that setting goals in 90-day increments will significantly raise your productivity.

Start here: *Financial Success with the YL90 Plan.*

Dear Carrie & Elena,

After my second child was born, I used to stay up late into the night trying to catch up on all the things I never got to during the day. For a whole year I only slept about 4-5 hours each night. The next morning I took several ounces of NingXia Red and Multigreen capsules. That combo gave me energy and also kept me from getting sick. I was very thankful for the energy, nutrition and immune support I received from these supplements during a time when I had so much going on. I don't recommend subsisting on so little sleep, but sometimes in life it does happen and it's good to know that help is available.

—Kyong P. NJ

"Concentrate all your thoughts upon the work at hand.
The sun's rays do not burn until brought to a focus."

—Alexander Graham Bell—

| Suggested Reading | *Releasing Emotional Patterns with Essential Oils -* Paperback by Carolyn L. Mein (Sept. 1, 1998) | *Feelings Buried Alive Never Die* by Karol Kuhn Truman (Paperback, Aug 1, 1991) |

Gallbladder / Liver

From detoxification to metabolism, the liver and gallbladder play key roles in digestion, cleansing, and providing nourishment. If the liver is not functioning at a high level, nutrients will not be absorbed efficiently.

. . . .

Tip: Since most gallstones are composed of cholesterol, diet plays a role in their formation. Try this: increase fiber, and vitamin C, drink more water, lose weight slowly, & limit your sugar intake.
—Dr. Andrew Weil.

. . . .

Our Approach:

Apply: Two drops of *JuvaCleanse* and **GLF** over the liver (across the abdomen) 2 times daily, warm compresses may be added as well.

Try: Two ounces of **NingXia Red** and 2-4 drops of *JuvaCleanse* in a capsule daily and **Super C** tablets.

Diffuse: *Thieves* daily to keep your home and office environment clean. The liver serves as a filter for toxins air-born and ingested. The less the liver has to process the healthier you will be.

Did you know?

Although the liver can be partially removed and the gallbladder removed completely due to serious illness, keeping them healthy and strong should be paramount and surgery avoided whenever possible.

Most toxins, or poisons, reach our bloodstream when we swallow or inhale them. Others pass through our skin, while still others are released by dying cells or invading bacteria. Many of these toxins pass through the liver -- the body's waste-purification plant -- where they are broken down and removed from the blood before they can do their dirty work. —Laurie Barclay, MD.

Essential oils are amazing detoxifiers. Whether applied, diffused, or ingested, these mighty oils are capable of eliminating the bad and avoiding the good. Knowing how best to use your oils, and when to use them, can be easily learned through the YL90 Plan brochure, *Essential Oil Basics*. Share these wonderful detoxifiers with your friends and family. Their livers will thank you for it!

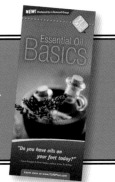

Dear Carrie & Elena,

To begin my liver cleanse I used Peppermint & Purification over my liver. They were my companion oils and extremely helpful.

I applied JuvaCleanse topically 1-2 times daily over my liver vita flex points & directly on my stomach for about 30 days. At the same time, I began taking JuvaTone 2 times per day & added JuvaFlex to my topical applications of JuvaCleanse 1-2 times daily.

After the cleanse I felt it was essential that I reintroduce good quality foods & supplements into my daily routine since I had just spent all this time detoxifying. I use Master Formula Hers, Super Cal, Ningxia Red, OmegaGize & Longevity.

I find all the Young Living products (cleansing & otherwise) to be very subtle & gentle, yet highly effective. All my systems are working really well now and 2 separate doctors of mine even said they wish they had a blood panel like mine!

—Jason W., Shine Yoga Center, NJ

"Old age is when the liver spots show through your gloves."

—Phyllis Diller—

| **Suggested Reading** | *Raindrop Technique* by D. Gary Young (Paperback, June 2008) | *The Complete Book of Essential Oils and Aromatherapy: Over 600 Natural, Non-Toxic and Fragrant Recipes to Create Health - Beauty - a Safe Home Environment* by Valerie Ann Worwood (Paperback, 1991) | *The Reference Guide to Essential Oils* (Softcover, 12th Edition, July 2010) |
| | *Ultimate Balance* by LeAnne Deardeuff, DC (Spiral bound, Apr. 2009) | | |

Hair Care

Some of the most toxic products on the market today are found in haircare products. Because we wash our hair often and sometimes apply many products to our hair and scalp, we are putting our health at risk if we are not aware of the ingredients we are putting on our head.

. . . . . .

Tip: Try this to avoid lice: In a 4 oz. bottle filled with water add 5 drops each of **Rosemary**, **Orange**, and **Peppermint**, shake well each time before using. Spray on hair daily before going out. It can also be sprayed on clothes, coats, bedding, & plush toys.

. . . . . .

Our Approach:

Use: *Lavender Mint Shampoo & Conditioner* in the spring/summer or if hair is oily to normal and *Copaiba Vanilla Shampoo & Conditioner* in the fall/winter or if hair is normal to dry. Use very little of each (they are very concentrated) and rinse thoroughly.

Try: *Core Supplements*, *Sulfurzyme* capsules, and **NingXia Red** daily. Feeding you body well will also yield strong, beautiful hair.

Apply: A small amount of *Animal Scents Ointment* to dry hair over night for deep conditioning. Shampoo and Condition as usual in the morning. Used sparingly, *Animals Scents Ointment* can be used to style your hair and keep hair in place, and gets rid of "fly aways."

Did you know?

Gentle cleansing agents derived from sources like coconut, nuts, and palm oil bring foam, spreadability, and a deeper clean into the shower. (Coconut derivatives are the most popular cleansers. On labels, seek out words with "coco" or "cocyl" in the ingredients list.) When you lather up with a natural shampoo, add water to generate extra foam instead of slopping on more product. Because they're made with oils adding more shampoo adds more oil to the scalp, leaving hair limp.

The change of seasons and outdoor activities can be especially damaging and stressful to the hair. From swimming to sunstress, your hair certainly takes a beating in the summer. Avoid harmful ingredients such as sodium laurel sulfate and any type of paraben.

Use our haircare tips in the YL90 Plan brochure, *The Great Outdoors*, to keep hair looking great all year round. Our brochure also contains beauty secrets for great skin.

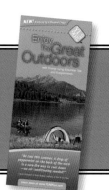

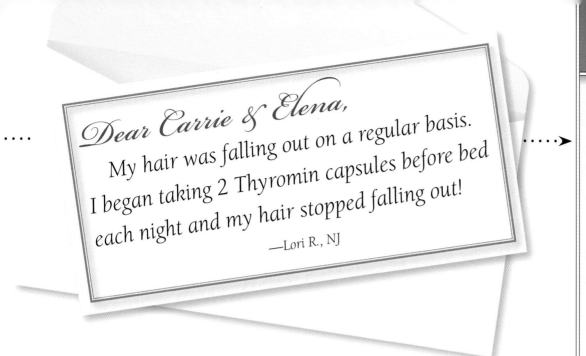

Dear Carrie & Elena,

My hair was falling out on a regular basis. I began taking 2 Thyromin capsules before bed each night and my hair stopped falling out!

—Lori R., NJ

"Beauty isn't worth thinking about; what's important is your mind. You don't want a fifty-dollar haircut on a fifty-cent head."

—Garrison Keillor—

Suggested Reading

Aromatherapy for Dummies by Kathi Keville (Paperback, Sept 15, 1999)

500 Formulas For Aromatherapy: Mixing Essential Oils for Every Use by Carol Schiller and David Schiller (Paperback, June 30, 1994)

Aromatherapy Handbook for Beauty, Hair, and Skin Care by Erich Keller (Paperback, Sept. 1, 1999)

Headaches

From a dull nagging pain to debilitating migraines, headaches are very common. Knowing the source of your headache will help you use your essential oils more effectively. Treatment for a sinus headache may differ from one caused by stress or hormone imbalance.

. . . .

Tip: Many times, you can prevent the onset of migraines by providing sufficient nutrients to your body that help prevent blood vessel constriction. —*Psychology Today*. Also see the "Try" section at right.

. . . .

Our Approach:

Apply: One to two drops of **PanAway**, **Aroma Siez**, or **M-Grain** to the temples and the back of the neck.

Try: **BLM** and **Sulfurzyme** *capsules* in combination with *2 ounces of* **NingXia Red** daily. Also take a **Super B** tablet at night.

Diffuse: **Peppermint** or **Basil** during your headache. Take 15 minutes to lie down and breathe.

Did you know?

"Therapeutic essential oils from Young Living like **Idaho Tansy** *and* **Roman Chamomile** *may help enhance the oxygen carrying capacity of the blood and oxygen infusion into the cell according to the Essential Oils Desk Reference as compiled by Life Science Publishing."* —Joseph Mercola, DO

For women only:

Many headaches are rooted in hormonal imbalances. **Progessence Plus** drops applied topically, 2 times daily, is an easy solution for many women who suffer from migraines. The results can take time. Hormone balancing can take 6-8 weeks to take effect. Don't despair if you don't see results immediately. We always recommend sticking to something for at least 90-days.

Headaches have many root causes and are often difficult to diagnose. No matter what the cause of the pain, essential oils can have a positive effect on eliminating and preventing pain. Our basic pain relief program in the YL90 Plan brochure, *Live Pain Free*, can help to adjust your body's natural ability to reduce inflammation and minimize headaches.

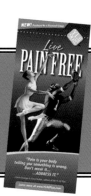

SINGLES:
  Basil
  Idaho Tansy
  Peppermint
  Roman Chamomile

OIL BLENDS:
  Aroma Siez
  M-Grain
  PanAway

SUPPLEMENTS:
  BLM
  NingXia Red
  Sulfurzyme
  Super B

PERSONAL CARE:
  Progessence Plus

Dear Carrie & Elena,

I have suffered from migraines since I was a teenager. I would have migraines sometimes 2 or 3 times per month that would cause me to be nauseous. When over the counter pain and headache medication did not help any more my doctor switched me to prescription pain medication that only worked when taken at the very start of a migraine.

I then tried using Basil essential oil. I put 2 drops on the brain stem (top of the spine at the back of my neck) and massage it in over a minute. The migraine goes away. I can use it at any time during the migraine. In extreme cases I re-apply within an hour or two.

—Christine G., NJ

"A great wind is blowing, and that gives you either imagination or a headache."

—Catherine the Great—

Suggested Reading	*Healing With Aromatherapy* by Marlene Ericksen (Jun 15, 2000)	*What Your Doctor May Not Tell You About Migraines* by Alexander Mauskop, M.D., and Barry Fox, Ph.D. (Paperback, 2001)

Heart Health

The heart is considered the "center" of our emotions but it is also vital to our overall health and longevity. Taking care of your heart means eating well, getting plenty of rest, and daily exercise.

. . . .

Tip: Good circulation will put less stress on the heart. Massage your legs and arms with *Cypress* oil to promote good circulation, especially the hands and feet.

. . . .

Our Approach:

Apply: *Peace & Calming* and *Aroma Life* over the heart 1-2 times daily if you are dealing with a cardiovascular problem or a chronic condition. To support your heart on a regular basis try to repeat 1-2 times a week.

Try: *OmegaGize* and *Longevity capsules* and 2 ounces *NingXia Red*, daily. We also like taking *Mineral Essence* drops and *Essentialzyme* capsules in addition to the above supplements for extra support.

Diffuse: *Peace & Calming* to reduce stress.

Did you know?

Every organ in the body -- especially the heart, muscles, and kidneys -- needs the mineral magnesium. It also contributes to the makeup of teeth and bones. Most important, it activates enzymes, contributes to energy production, and helps regulate calcium levels as well as copper, zinc, potassium, vitamin D, and other important nutrients in the body. —Live Strong

Exercise does not have to be demanding or stressful. Take a walk everyday and you will see a drop in your weight and improvement in your heart health. Exercise and a healthy weight provides an excellent foundation for heart health.

Coronary heart disease, high blood pressure, stroke, heart attacks & angina can all be brought on by the disruption of hormone balance caused by synthetic hormones found in foods, medicines, birth control or personal care products.

Balancing your hormones naturally can help support a healthy heart.

Follow our tips in the YL90 Plan brochure, *Healthy Woman: Hormone Rescue Guide.*

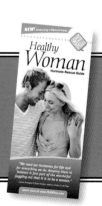

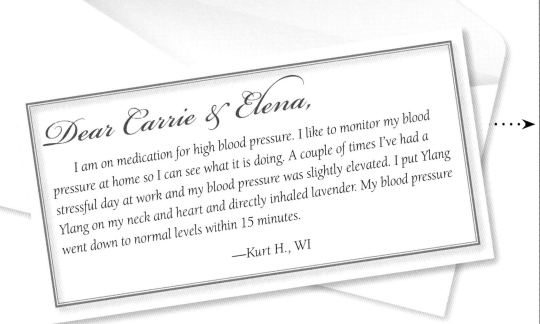

Dear Carrie & Elena,

I am on medication for high blood pressure. I like to monitor my blood pressure at home so I can see what it is doing. A couple of times I've had a stressful day at work and my blood pressure was slightly elevated. I put Ylang Ylang on my neck and heart and directly inhaled lavender. My blood pressure went down to normal levels within 15 minutes.

—Kurt H., WI

Peter, an 82 year old man, went to the doctor for a full physical check-up. A few days later the doctor saw Peter walking through the village with a stunning young woman on his arm.

The doctor spoke to Peter quietly, but clearly, "You're really doing well aren't you?

Peter smiled happily, "Oh yes, but I'm only doing what you said Doc, "Get a hot mamma and be cheerful."

The doctor grimaced and retorted, "I didn't say that Peter, I said, You've got a heart murmur, be careful!"

Suggested Reading

Reversing Heart Disease: A Vital New Program to Help Prevent, Treat, and Eliminate Cardiac Problems Without Surgery by Julian M. Whitaker (Mar 1, 2002)

Lower Your Blood Pressure in Eight Weeks: A Revolutionary Program for a Longer, Healthier Life by Stephen T. Sinatra (Feb 4, 2003)

The New 8-Week Cholesterol Cure by Robert Kowalski (Oct 31, 2006)

Immune Support

Your best defense against any illness is a strong immune system. The Immune system is constantly changing, trying to stay ahead of everything that attacks our bodies. Providing support to this system should be a daily pursuit.

. . . .

Tip: Vitamin C tops the list of immune boosters for many reasons. There has been more research about the immune-boosting effects of Vitamin C than perhaps any other nutrient. —Dr. Sears

. . . .

Our Approach:

Apply: One to two drops of *Thieves* to the bottom of the feet once or twice a day, 6 days a week, in the fall/winter months and apply 1-2 drops of *Purification* or *Melrose* to the bottom of the feet once or twice a day, 6 days a week, in the spring/summer. We like to take a day off from our oil and supplement routine each week. When illness does strike, add *Immupower* to the above 3 oils on the feet and spine every two hours.

Try: *Inner Defense* and *Super C*, drink 2 ounces of *NingXia Red* during the day and a *Life 5* capsule at night before bed.

Diffuse: *Thieves* and *Purification*.

Did you know?

The greatest advantage an essential oil has over something that is man-made is its ability to quickly adapt to its surroundings. Just like a bacteria can turn into a "super bug", an essential oil can adapt to the germ it's fighting. Vaccines, antibiotics, and other medicines are created "as is" and cannot adapt or change to fit a situation. If the germ gets ahead of your medicine, the germ will win every time. On the other hand, medicinal plants keep coming back, stronger and smarter.

Get your defense system ready. Start a 90-day plan to a stronger immune system with the YL90 Plan brochure, *Essential Oil Basics*.

Applying, ingesting, and diffusing essential oils will not only help stimulate but will be absorbed through all three parts of the immune system—the skin, digestion, and respiratory system giving you the power to attack the things that attack you.

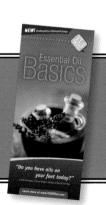

Dear Carrie & Elena,

During cold and flu season, I diffuse Thieves oil every day for at least an hour. I make sure my whole family is in the room while I do this, so we all get the benefit.

I also apply Thieves oil to everyone's feet each night before bed, and every morning to the kids' feet before they go to school. If I feel a scratchy throat coming on, I take a few Inner Defense capsules before bed and drink 3-4 ounces of NingXia Red with a drop of lemon oil.

Usually by the next morning, the scratchy throat is gone and I've avoided the infection by giving my immune system that extra boost to fight the germs.

—Justin G., NJ

Dr Kathleen Holloway of the World Health Organization (WHO) told CNN that antibiotic resistance is a global problem, with diseases including childhood pneumonia, dysentery and tuberculosis (TB) no longer responding to first-line antibiotics in some parts of the world.

"Every human being is the author of his own health or disease."
—Buddha—

Suggested Reading *What to Do When Antibiotics Don't Work! How to Stay Healthy and Alive When Infections Strike* by Dirk Van Gils (Paperback, July 3, 2002)

Encyclopedia of Natural Medicine, Revised Second Edition by Michael Murray and Joseph Pizzorno (Dec 29, 1997)

Kidney / Bladder

Produced by the kidneys and eliminated through the bladder, urine contains the byproducts of metabolism — salts, toxins, and water. It is the way the body gets rid of waste that would end up in the blood.

. . . .

Tip: *Juniper* and *Tangerine* are natural diuretics. If you find that you need to reduce fluid in the body, try these natural solutions and drink plenty of water. The minerals in the water keep the body from becoming too dehydrated.

. . . .

Our Approach:

Apply: One to two drops of **Nutmeg**, **Sandalwood**, and **Juniper** to the lower back.

Try: **K&B Tincture** drops in capsules and 2 ounces of **NingXia Red** daily.

Diffuse: **Thieves** in the air to put less stress on the body.

Did you know?

The National Association For Continence (NAFC) reports about 25 million adult Americans experience transient or chronic problems with urinary incontinence—and the vast majority who struggle with passing urine accidentally, around 75 percent, are women.

According to the Mayo Clinic web site, the major types of medications used to relieve urinary incontinence are anticholinergics, alpha-adrenergic agonists and estrogen. All these drugs are laden with potential side effects ranging from dry mouth, dizziness, constipation, heartburn, blurry vision and urinary retention to impaired memory, confusion and even cancer.

Supplements help to rest the kidneys in order to allow them to recover, repair and function optimally once more. A delicate balance of diet, fluids, supplements and exercise are needed in order to repair the kidneys and provide the rest that the kidneys need to repair them for a long and healthy future. —Natural News, February 2009.

Women often suffer from kidney and bladder infections. Supporting the kidneys early in puberty can help a woman strengthen her kidneys and bladder to prevent infections from occurring.

Getting your hormones working properly goes a long way in supporting other systems of the body, too.

Try our YL90 Plan, *Healthy Woman: Hormone Rescue Guide* to put your body on the right track.

SINGLES:

Juniper
Nutmeg
Sandalwood
Tangerine

OIL BLENDS:

Thieves

SUPPLEMENTS:

K & B Tincture
NingXia Red

Dear Carrie & Elena,

I introduced K&B to clean my kidneys. I did this for 8 days. (K&B is an incredible product. having suffered for many years with recurring urinary tract infections it felt great to cleanse my kidneys & bladder). I also find that drinking about 3 drops of Thieves oil in 6-8 oz. water, chased with another 16 oz. of pure water also helps to flush the system for maintenance.

—Tracy R, Shine Yoga Center, NJ

"*But I know all about love already. I know precious little about kidneys.*"

—Aldous Huxley—

| Suggested Reading | *Essential Oils Desk Reference,* Fifth Edition by Gary Young (2011) | *The Complete Book of Essential Oils and Aromatherapy: Over 600 Natural, Non-Toxic and Fragrant Recipes to Create Health - Beauty - a Safe Home Environment* by Valerie Ann Worwood (1991) | *Living Balanced:* Stacey A. Kimbrell (Paperback, 2009) |

Libido

Our libido is a combination of the mind and body. Sex drive can be effected by a number of factors such as hormones, family, work, age, medications, stress, and more.

. . . .

Tip: Enjoying an active sex life is essential to our well being, and the foods we eat play a large role in ensuring we feel sexy. Some of the foods that help turn us on include: pumpkin seeds, avocados, bee pollen, and figs; supplements containing these foods include **NingXia Red**, **Mineral Essence**, & **Super Cal**.

. . . .

Our Approach:

Apply: One drop *Sandalwood, Jasmine, Rose, Ylang Ylang, Sensation,* or *Live with Passion* to pulse points or those of your partner; dilute generously with V6 Mixing Oil on sensitive areas.

Try: *OmegaGize* and *Longevity* capsules as directed; drink 2 oz. of *NingXia Red*, daily.

Diffuse: *Sensation* or *Jasmine* to set the mood.

Did you know?

Essential oils can be very effective in stimulating the libido.

Sandalwood has been known since ancient times to improve blood flow, balance mood, and stimulate interest. Because its scent is close to a man's, it is especially effective for women.

Jasmine is known to tame anger, raise interest, and inspire passion.

Ylang Ylang, jasmine's close counterpart, is less expensive and has similar properties.

Rose, perhaps the most expensive and rare is also one of the most effective. From Cleopatra to Snow White, rose is associated with love, passion, and romance.

All four of these oils can be diffused or applied. They can also be added to **V6 Mixing Oil** to make a massage oil.

Balancing your hormones is key to having a healthy libido. Whether you are young or old, supporting your hormones is necessary. Your libido can change over time with fluctuating hormones. Maintainaing a healthy level with an over-all hormone balancer like PD 80/20 capsules is a good place to start.

For more helpful tips follow our suggestion in the YL90 Plan brochure, *Healthy Woman: Hormone Rescue Guide.*

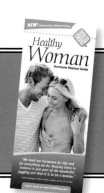

Dear Carrie & Elena,

I love the Sensation products – especially the oil and bath gel! After a long day at work and conflicting schedules (not to mention kids and aging parents living in the same household) it can be a challenge to find time to be alone when you're "in the mood". Sensation is a great way to send a signal to your beloved that tonight's the night.

—Xorti Y., NJ

"Sex appeal is fifty percent what you've got and fifty percent what people think you've got."

—Sophia Loren—

| **Suggested Reading** | *Healthy Sex Drive, Healthy You: What Your Libido Reveals About Your Life* by Dr. Diana Hoppe, (Paperback, April 1, 2010)

Aroma: The International Magazine for Essential Oils. Nr. 1/Winter 2000: Lavender, by Terra Linda Scent and Image Inc. (Hardcover, 2000) | *Sensational Sex in 7 Easy Steps: The Proven Plan for Enhancing Your Sexual Function and Achieving Optimum Health* by Ridwan Shabsigh, MD, Bruce Scali, Dr. Mehmet Oz. (Paperback, Mar 6, 2007) |

Men's Health

Beginning a regimen of supplements, whole foods, and essential oils may protect you from ailments that are common to men. Making small changes can have a great effect on your health, longevity, and strength at any age. You are your own best caretaker.

· · · · · · ·

Tip: The essential oils in *Prostate Health* contain key anti-inflammatory components that, combined with saw palmetto and pumpkin seed oil, help fight cancer and protect prostate function. (*Super B* and *Longevity* are great complementary products.)

· · · · · · ·

Our Approach:

Apply: *Mister* to the ankles, starting with a couple of drops once a week slowly increasing until you feel that your hormones are balanced. Apply *Abundance* or *Valor* daily instead of chemically based colognes and aftershave products.

Try: *Master Formula His* vitamins, *OmegaGize* capsules, a *Super* B tablet, a *Longevity* capsule, and drink 2 oz. of **NingXia Red**, daily. To strengthen your bones, ligaments, and muscles, add **BLM** capsules.

Diffuse: *Peace & Calming* to reduce stress. *Clarity* or *En-R-Gee* to increase productivity at home or at the office.

Did you know?

Men often feel like they have to hold up the world; allowing the stress of family and work to come before their health, until a crisis occurs.

Here are some of the active ingredients in the natural supplements listed in the "Try" section above:

Calcium & vitamin D: to maintain a healthy weight and strengthen bones;
Chromium: to ward off diabetes;
Folic acid: to fight against Alzheimer's and Parkinson's diseases;

Glucosamine: to grease your joints;
Omega-3: to protect your heart;
Selenium: to fight cancer; and
Vitamin E: to slow aging.

Don't feel overwhelmed by thought the of adding a healthy regimen to your life. Simple steps can be easily taken following the YL90 Plan's brochure, *Essential Oil Basics*.

Learning how to use natural products is as easy as 1-2-3—apply, diffuse, ingest. Follow our guide and in 90 days you'll feel a difference—and want to share that difference with a friend. Our brochure is better than a business card, it's a one-stop shop for all you need to get started.

OIL BLENDS:

Abundance
Clarity
En-R-Gee
Mister
Peace & Calming
Valor

SUPPLEMENTS:

BLM
Longevity
Master Formula His
NingXia Red
OmegaGize
Prostate Health
Super B

Dear Carrie & Elena,

I'm a college student and by far, my favorite oil is Peppermint; I put it in my coffee or tea to wake me up in the morning. I also use Valor on my feet because it gives me a boost for my day and makes me more focused during my work out.

But my best recommendation for essential oils is Lavender for poison ivy. My father, brother and I were clearing out wooded trails for a hunting club using a chain saw. As we were cutting the underbrush and small trees, the oil from the poison ivy plant became airborne and went not just on my skin but into my lungs. When the rash developed, the itching was unbearable and went on for days. I used a topical steroid cream and then was given steroid pills which made me act very angrily and out of character.

I started taking 1 or 2 drops of Lavender oil in an 8oz. glass of water and the itching went away fast. I was in an incredible amount of discomfort, and the Lavender was like a miracle drug! After the extreme itching had gone on for so many days, the Lavender took it out in fifteen minutes flat.

I drank a glass of water with Lavender oil whenever the itching would come back (about every 2 hours at first). I heard later that oil in capsules would work well too. After about a week the itching went away and never came back.

—Nick O., VA

"With self-discipline most anything is possible."

—Theodore Roosevelt—

Suggested Reading

The Men's Health Big Book of Food and Nutrition by Joel Weber and Mike Zimmerman (Paperback, Dec. 21 2010)

A New Route to Robust Health - by D. Gary Young (Paperback, 2000)

The Harvard Medical School Guide to Men's Health: Lessons from the Harvard Men's Health Study by Harvey B. Simon (Paperback, Feb. 3, 2004)

Sensational Sex in 7 Easy Steps: The Proven Plan for Enhancing Your Sexual Function and Achieving Optimum Health (Paperback, 2007)

Nausea, Vomiting, Upset Stomach

Nausea, vomiting, or upset stomach is our body's way of ridding itself of toxins. When we digest our foods our immune system slows down. Not eating heavily allows the immune system to kick into gear. So listen to your body when these symptoms strike.

· · · · · · ·

Tip: Essential oils can be put in a cup of warm water and consumed like tea or put into a warm bath. But remember, If it's too hot for you to drink or bathe in, then it's too hot for the oil. Heating oils at extremely high temperatures may damage the oil. Warm water is also easier for the body to assimilate.

· · · · · · ·

Our Approach:

Apply: *Ginger*, *Peppermint*, or *Di-Gize* to the abdomen, back and feet.

Try: *Ginger*, *Peppermint*, or *Di-Gize* in a glass of water or a drop or two in a capsule. Sip the water slowly. Drinking too much water can encourage vomiting.

Diffuse: Or inhale *Ginger*, *Peppermint*, or *Di-Gize*.

Did you know?

Can't stand to drink anything? Try making an ice cube with a drop of essential oil. A little goes a long way so you may want to add a drop of *Peppermint* to a pitcher of water (mix well with a whisk and pour immediately, as the oil tends to float to the top) and then fill your ice tray. This not only helps to flavor cool drinks but you can suck on the ice cube when you are sick which may be easier to tolerate than a full glass of water.

The essential oil of *Ginger* is an essential in your herbal arsenal for nausea. *Ginger* is widely used for digestive issues of all types as it improves digestion, calms nausea, encourages gastric juices to form and has countless other digestive benefits. Through scent, essential oils can travel to the limbic system of your brain, which responds by releasing neurotransmitters and hormones. Essential oils also work by absorption through the skin into the blood stream. —*LiveStrong.com*

Nausea may be only one of the many symptoms you are experiencing when ill. What can start off as an upset stomach can turn into fever, cough, runny nose and more overnight.

Having the YL90 Plan brochure, *Cold-N-Flu fighters* and having the oils recommended in the brochure on hand will insure that you are prepared when nausea and other illness strike. Don't get caught without the products and the plan that you need.

Dear Carrie & Elena,

We JUST experienced a stomach flu at my house. Of all times for it to hit... it hit my 4 year old in the car on Easter! I don't know HOW we escaped getting it, but my 2 year old, my husband, and I (pregnant) have avoided it.

I had Thieves spray in the car with me and sprayed everything in the car that I could... including my hands and mouth. That night, I was up with my son who was vomiting almost every hour. The times he went the longest between vomiting was after I'd apply peppermint and Di-Gize to his belly and feet. (Dilute those on the belly for kids and adults). I diffused Thieves in his room, and ImmuPower in the house for the rest of us. I kept spraying EVERYTHING with diluted Thieves Cleaner, including the toys and kids' hands. We also did LOTS of hand washing.

I opened a Life 5 capsule and poured some into water to have my son drink. I figured he'd absorb something before he vomited it up. I gave it to him right after he vomited to allow for the longest time to absorb before the next cycle. I kept him well hydrated, and had him sip water frequently.

The next day I began to use ImmuPower, Oregano, and Clove on his feet. He had a bad fever for 2 days with a headache, body aches, and stiff neck, so I used Wintergreen, PanAway, and Peppermint frequently to help him feel better. I applied the Peppermint to his forehead, neck, and feet.

For me, I had been absorbing the oils through my hands from applying them to my son, so I didn't go crazy in taking them myself. I did spray my mouth occasionally with the Thieves spray, and I did use Oregano specifically on my feet. We all drank NingXia Red (except for the sick one who would've just puked it up).

Good luck and feel better to anyone who reads this!

—Kerry, S. NJ

Shopping List

SINGLES:
Ginger
Peppermint

OIL BLENDS:
Di-Gize

> "By swallowing evil words unsaid, no one has ever harmed his stomach."
>
> —Winston Churchill—

Suggested Reading *The Complete Book of Essential Oils and Aromatherapy: Over 600 Natural, Non-Toxic and Fragrant Recipes to Create Health - Beauty - a Safe Home Environment* by Valerie Ann Worwood (Paperback, 1991)

The Aromatherapy Bible: The Definitive Guide to Using Essential Oils by Gill Farrer-Halls (Paperback, Aug. 1, 2005)

Nutrition

Nothing is a better friend to nutrition than an essential oil. Combine an essential oil with a whole food or a whole food supplement and you have a powerful health tool.

· · · · · · ·

Tip: Have fun with your food and take it to go! Making clean, whole foods at home and carrying them in fun containers like a bento box and treating yourself to a "fun" condiment like lemon wedges, wasabi, salsa, or citrus oil can help to break up monotony.

· · · · · · ·

Our Approach:

Apply: Your favorite essential oils to your feet daily. We like *Thieves* & *Valor*. All essential oils will help with the absorption of nutrients.

Try: *Core Supplements*, which include: *Longevity, OmegaGize , Life 5, and True Source.* For antioxidant support drink 2 oz. of *NingXia Red* daily.

Diffuse: *Citrus Fresh*, *Peace & Calming*, or *Pine* essential oils can be absorbed through inhalation as well as application and ingestion. Coniferous oils can help oxygenate the blood increasing nutritional absorption.

Did you know?

The "SAD or Standard American Diet" is significantly lacking in key nutrients. What's worse is that processed foods are filled with preservatives, salt and sugars (refined and artificial), which can be addicting and contain empty calories. Getting on a whole-food supplementation program and a "clean eating" diet is one way to break the cycle of food addiction and sluggish metabolism.

Eating cleanly means you don't have to count calories. Clean foods like whole fruits and vegetables, whole grains, nuts, seeds, lean meats, eggs, and fish have very few calories yet are packed with nutrition. Avoid foods loaded with calories and void of nutrition. Watch portion sizes.

One way to increase your nutrition is to get rid of toxins that have built up in our fat. Essential oils and oil enhanced supplements are very effective in burning fats and releasing toxins.

Citrus oils have been know for years as fat burners. Learn how to use these and other oils and supplements to get rid of toxins and increase nutrition.

Follow our easy guide in the YL90 Plan, *Fat Loss That Works.*

Dear Carrie & Elena,

I am the owner of a busy spa where many people come for restorative treatments. I encourage them to eat healthily between visits because I know that it will support whatever healing they have experienced and rebuild the spirit. Essential oils added to foods can provide the added "oomph" or "umami" that make a dish delicious and stimulating to all the basic senses of taste: sweet, salty, bitter, sour. On my blog I frequently add a recipe that is seasonal. Here is one that I have published in my "Restorative Recipes" column – Enjoy!

Use your essential oils in a healthy, fun way. Replace Gatorade with a cool mixture of oils.

Gatorade Replacement Ingredients:

2 oz. NingXia Red

16 oz. water

1 drop of Lemon oil

1 drop of Peppermint oil

1 teaspoon of Blue Agave

—Karin J., AcuSource Healing, NJ

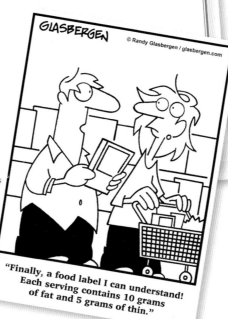

GLASBERGEN

© Randy Glasbergen / glasbergen.com

"Finally, a food label I can understand! Each serving contains 10 grams of fat and 5 grams of thin."

Shopping List

SINGLES:

Lemon
Pine

OIL BLENDS:

Citrus Fresh
Peace & Calming
Thieves
Valor

SUPPLEMENTS:

Core Supplements
Longevity
NingXia Red
OmegaGize
Life 5
True Source

Suggested Reading

Food Rules: An Eater's Manual by Michael Pollan (Dec 29, 2009)

The Omnivore's Dilemma: A Natural History of Four Meals by Michael Pollan (Aug 28, 2007)

The Eat-Clean Diet: Fast Fat-Loss that lasts Forever! by Tosca Reno (Jan 8, 2007)

Green Smoothie Revolution: The Radical Leap Towards Natural Health by Victoria Boutenko (Aug 4, 2009)

The Raw Food Feast: 7 Days Through the Rainbow by Mandilyn Canistelle (Paperback, 2010)

Pain Relief

Pain can strike when we are not expecting it and can seem to last with no end in sight. Fighting the root cause of your pain is key to relief. Essential oils are effective because they go right to work at the cellular level.

· · · · · · ·

Tip: Try these different applications of essential oils to alleviate pain: in warm baths, compresses or full body massage. Oils like *Valor* applied before or during acupuncture, yoga, or chiropractic adjustments can enhance the effect of these modalities.

· · · · · · ·

Our Approach:

Apply: To the area of pain a few drops of: *PanAway*, *Aroma Siez*, *Deep Relief*, and/or *Relieve It* (singly or in any combination). For a full body massage apply *OrthoEase* and/or *OrthoSport* (of the two, *OrthoSport* is stronger). Add any of the first three oil blends listed to the *OrthoEase* or *OrthoSport* for added relief on large areas. For joint pain and pain associated with chronic illness or hormone imbalance, try *Regenolone Cream*.

Try: Drink 1-2 oz. of *NingXia Red* and take *BLM* capsules, and *Sulfurzyme* capsules as directed, twice daily.

Diffuse: *Peace & Calming*, *Lavender*, or other calming oil. Tension and stress can exacerbate pain. Relaxation can be the first step to pain relief.

Did you know?

You are never too old to relieve pain. "I am an 80 year old woman and have suffered pain in my joints for 40 years. Although I tried many drugs, the side effects were terrible. Now I use an essential oil recipe for pain. I apply *Cypress*, *Wintergreen*, and *Balsam Fir* where I feel pain, morning and night.

I have also had two knee surgeries. I used PanAway topically with great success for pain and scaring. I took a capsule with 2-3 drops each of *Helichrysum*, *Wintergreen*, *Frankincense*, and *Copaiba* to help manage the pain for a year after surgery." —Clara O., NY

The YL90 Plan, *Live Pain Free*, takes a two-pronged approach; oils and supplements. We find that using the two in combination is the winning formula.

Pain is best defeated when attacked both from the inside and outside.

Make a commitment and be consistent. Keep up with the program for at least 90 days to get the results you want.

Dear Carrie & Elena,

I was in a horrible car accident with an 18-wheeler at 55 MPR. Lying on the highway, I found the strength to ask for my essential oil bag so I could apply Tranquil Roll-on and Stress Away Roll-on. The ambulance came and I was rushed to a Trauma Unit. My dear friend, Lillian, was called and she came with a bag full of oils. My left leg and knee were severely swollen, bruised and inflamed. My chest, arms, sternum, and back were killing me from the airbag. I was unable to move my arms and could not sit up at all.

We immediately started to pour oils on my leg and chest. - PanAway, Deep Relief, Frankincense, Helichrysum and Lavender and massaged into the area. We applied Stress Away Roll-on and Sacred Frankincense to my wrists and forehead. Lillian had brought a NingXia Red pack to the hospital and when I was able to drink, that was the first thing I drank. Nothing was broken and they sent me home.

The first few days were very painful and I was wary about taking any prescription drugs for the pain. So I use the oils every hour: applied: 2 drops of each: Helichrysum, Lavender, Frankincense, Copaiba, PanAway and Deep Relief Roll-on; ingested: 1 drop frankincense, 1 drop Copaiba, 1 drop Lavender and 1 drop Wintergreen every 2 hours; drank: 6-8 oz. of NingXia Red a day. After 3 days... applied: 2 drops Balsam Fir, 2 drops Copaiba and 2 drops Lavender and instead of taking vegetable capsules of oils, I added 2 drops Frankincense, 2 drops Copaiba and 2 drops of peppermint to 2 ounces of NingXia Red.

On the third day I started back to my meditation and yoga/breathing practices. I am feeling so much better and I am still sore but I know and believe that it the oils, yoga, and breathing are why I am back to teaching yoga and moving around so well. Thank you to all the angels in my life!

—Jan Jeremias, RYT, NJ. Aroma Lotus Yoga

Shopping List

SINGLES:

Balsam Fir
Copaiba
Cypress
Frankincense
Helichrysum
Lavender
Wintergreen

OIL BLENDS:

Aroma Siez
Deep Relief Roll-on
PanAway
Peace & Calming
Relieve It
Valor

SUPPLEMENTS:

BLM
NingXia Red
Sulfurzyme

PERSONAL CARE:

OrthoEase
OrthoSport
Regenolone Cream

| **Suggested Reading** | *Dr. Earl Mindell, The Power of MSM* by Earl L. Mindell, R.Ph., Ph.D, and Virginia Hopkins (Paperback, May 16, 2002) | *The Acid Alkaline Balance Diet* by Felicia Drury Kliment, (Paperback, 2002) | *The Miracle of MSM: The Natural Solution for Pain* by Stanley Jacob, M.D. (Paperback, Dec 13, 1999) |

Pregnancy

Using essential oils and supplements when pregnant or becoming pregnant is a personal choice that must be made with your spouse and medical advisor.

. . . .

Tip: Knowledge builds confidence and ability. Try eating mindfully and appreciatively (eating protein can reduce sugar cravings), move and play (improve posture), surround yourself with goodness (listen to those with a positive voice), dream (listen to yourself and what your body and soul are telling you). —*www.mothersnaturally.org*

. . . .

Our Approach:

Apply: The oil of your choice *diluted*. Even if you used to use an oil neat, your skin sensitivity can change during pregnancy and it's always best to be cautious. ***Lemon***, ***Lavender,*** and ***Gentle Baby*** are traditional favorites of moms-to-be.

Try: ***True Source*** vitamins or ***KidScents MightyVites*** multivitamins. You may find the kids vitamins easier to digest during pregnancy. Young Living's natural personal care product line of dental, hair, and skin care can help limit your exposure to toxins.

Diffuse: Or inhale ***Ginger***, ***Peppermint***, or ***Di-Gize*** to limit nausea.

Did you know?

Nerve cells or neurons are produced in the fetus at an average rate of 250,000 per minute.

Once you have seen a fetal heartbeat the risk of miscarriage lowers to 5%.

Unborn babies can feel, see and hear, so spend time stroking your belly and talking to your baby in the womb.

Every human spent an hour as a single cell. —*www.welcomebabyhome.com*

Learning how to use essential oils safely and in multiple arenas can become a useful life tool. Limiting the number of chemicals in personal care, medications, and cleaners will help to green your body, environment, and your family.

Follow the suggestions in the YL90 Plan, *Green Cleaning Solutions*, for tips on how to make your home safe, natural, and clean for you and your baby.

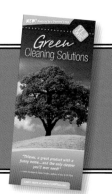

Dear Carrie & Elena,

I suffered from horrific nausea during both of my pregnancies, which lasted from the beginning until the baby was born. During my first pregnancy I tried everything anyone suggested. I drank more water, ate more protein, had salty crackers before I got up, drank tea, you name it. Nothing worked. It was so debilitating that I had to stop working (which isn't easy because I run my own business).

The second time around, I had been introduced to Young Living Oils already, and as soon as the intense nausea began, I used Peppermint and Lemon oils. I rubbed Peppermint oil on my belly and diffused Lemon oil. The results were unbelievable. I was able to function with them, but if I forgot to use them or bring them with me, I was in bad shape."

—Amara Wagner, www.amarawellness.com, NJ,

Every child begins the world again.

—Henry David Thoreau—

Suggested Reading

Gentle Babies: Essential Oils and Natural Remedies for Pregnancy, Childbirth, Infants and Young Children by Debra Raybern (Paperback, 2010)

Reference Guide for Esential Oils by Connie and Alan Higley, 12th edition (Spiral Bound, July 2010)

Aromatherapy and Massage for Mother and Baby by Allison England (Paperback, Nov 1, 2000)

Growing Healthy Families: Cooking with Holistic Moms by Holistic Moms Network, www.holisticmoms.org. (Paperback, Jan. 2000)

Skincare

The skin is the largest organ of the body. As part of the immune system it protects us from outside invaders, helps to regulate body temperature, and reflects our age and state of health. Take care of your skin, and your skin will take care of you.

· · · · · · ·

Tip: Wash off your make up at night! Make up not only contains harmful chemicals but will hold air pollutants to the skin causing pores to become clogged and damage the skin's surface. A clean face gives the body time to repair the skin while you sleep.

· · · · · · ·

Our Approach:

Apply: *ART Skin Care* products to your face. You can enhance the *ART* creams by adding either *Acne Skin Serum* or *Dry Skin Serum*. For your body choose "clean" bath gels, soaps, and lotions, avoiding the ingredients listed on the next page. Our favorites are: *Lavender Bath Gel*, *Valor Bar Soap*, *Thieves Hand Pump Soap*, and *Genesis Lotion*. Rinse with water and pat dry. Be sure to dampen the skin before washing. Applying a cleanser to dry skin can be harsh and is less effective. A drop of *Myrrh* applied to blemishes does the trick.

Try: Three *OmegaGize* capsules, drinking 1 oz. of *NingXia Red*, & taking 3 *Sulfurzyme* capsules, daily.

Diffuse: *Thieves* and *Purification* daily to kill air-born toxins that can effect the skin.

Did you know?

Face masks have been used since the time of Cleopatra. You can brighten your skin by combining a few simple ingredients. For dry skin mix equal parts unripened papaya, whole milk plain yogurt, and a few drops of *Geranium* oil. For oily skin mix equal parts avocado, cucumber, mineral rich green clay, and a few drops of Lemon oil. Apply either mask to the skin and allow to dry for 20 minutes. Rinse off with cool water and pat dry.

—WholeLiving.com

Many people battle skin allergies. From eczema to psoriasis these irritating and often painful conditions can attack children and adults alike.

Following our guide in the YL90 Plan brochure, *Allergies, Asthma, & Eczema*, will put you on a 90-day path to better skin. Don't give up. It takes time for the skin to heal. Be patient knowing that your skin is being supported with the right oils and supplements.

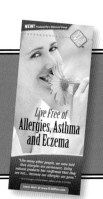

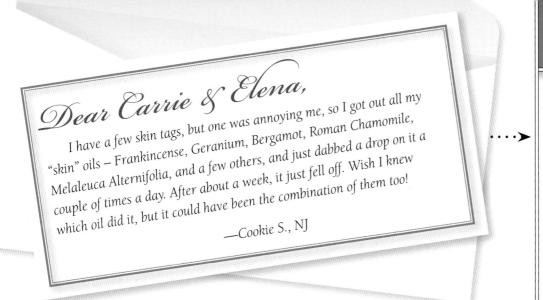

Dear Carrie & Elena,

I have a few skin tags, but one was annoying me, so I got out all my "skin" oils – Frankincense, Geranium, Bergamot, Roman Chamomile, Melaleuca Alternifolia, and a few others, and just dabbed a drop on it a couple of times a day. After about a week, it just fell off. Wish I knew which oil did it, but it could have been the combination of them too!

—Cookie S., NJ

Shopping List

SINGLES:

Myrrh
Geranium

OIL BLENDS:

Purification
Thieves

SUPPLEMENTS:

OmegaGize
NingXia Red
Sulfurzyme

PERSONAL CARE:

Acne Skin Serum
ART Skin Care
Dry Skin Serum
Genesis Lotion
Lavender Bath Gel
Thieves Hand
   Pump Soap
Valor Bar Soap

In her book, *Gorgeously Green*, Sophie Uliano recommends avoiding these ingredients in your skincare products: Parabens (methyl-, ethyl-, propyl-, butyl-, and isobutyl-), Fragrance, Polyethylene Glycol (PEG), Sodium Laurel Sulfate (SLS) and Sodium Lauryl Ether Sulfate (SLES),DEH, DEA, MEA, TEA & DEA, Quaternary Ammonium Compounds (Quats), Carbomer 934, 940, 941, 960, 961C, Talc.

As a white candle in a holy place, so is the beauty of an aged face.

-—Joseph Campbell—

Tanning beds are NOT safe!! Exposure to tanning beds before age 35 increases the risk of melanoma by 75%.

—University of Pennsylvania—

Suggested Reading

The Coconut Oil Miracle (Previously published as *The Healing Miracle of Coconut Oil*) by Bruce Fife and Jon J. Kabara (Paperback, Sept. 9, 2004)

The Essential Green You: Easy Ways to Detox Your Diet, Your Body, and Your Life by Deidre Imus. (Paperback, Dec. 3, 2008)

The New Guide to Remedies: Homeopathy; Essential Oils; Crystals; Home Remedies by Paragon Staff (Hardcover, 2005)

Sleeplessness

Whether your are stressed, sick, struggling with hormones, or depressed; sleeplessness can be hard to overcome, become chronic, and lead to many other health problems. Getting back on track quickly is vital to good health and wellbeing.

· · · · · · ·

Tip: Dr. Andrew Weil recommends **Valerian** and melatonin (in Sleepessence and ImmuPro) as the most well researched and trusted sleep aids of the natural world. Remember, the body responds better to complete darkness. Even the light from an alarm clock can interrupt sleep. Move small lights three feet from the bed.

· · · · · · ·

Our Approach:

Apply: (in order of strength) **Lavender**, **Tranquil Roll-on**, **Peace & Calming Roll-on**, **RutaVaLa**, or **Valerian**.

Try: One to two **ImmuPro** tablets or **Sleepessence** capsules. You can also put a drop of **Valerian** under your tongue. These products work within 20 minutes for most people.

Diffuse: Your favorite calming oil. We like **Lavender**, **Peace & Calming**, **Stress Away Roll-on**, **Orange**, or **Sacred Mountain**.

Did you know?

Coffee drinkers are far more likely to be poor sleepers. Caffeine and other dietary metabolic disrupters like MSG, sugar, white flour, and other carbohydrates make you think that you are "perking" up in the morning. In truth, they are actually disrupting your ability to sleep at night, even if these foods and drinks are only taken in the morning.

The main reason is their stress on your adrenal glands. In addition, your body's dependance on them will interrupt natural serotonin (the feel-good hormone) production. Without natural serotonin production we can become

What's troubling you? For most of us when we can't sleep it is our mind racing about unfinished issues or problems, or we find ourselves worrying because we can't sleep. Even emotional health can contribute to our ability to sleep.

Calming your stress can help you sleep soundly. Follow our easy oil and supplement suggestions in the YL90 Plan brochure, *End the Blues*, and have a good night's sleep.

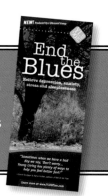

> ## Dear Carrie & Elena,
>
> My son had never been a great sleeper. It would take him approximately 45 minutes to 1 hour to stop the tossing & turning and finally go to sleep. After diffusing Peace & Calming for the first time, he fell asleep in 15 minutes. The next evening before bed he asked for his "nice smelly stuff". He fell asleep within 10 minutes. Since then, 4 years later, he has been sleeping with Peace & Calming diffusing every night on his nightstand.
>
> —Ann Linke, Linked with Holistic Health, GA

....

Shopping List

SINGLES:

Lavender
Nutmeg
Orange
Sandalwood
Valerian

OIL BLENDS:

Peace & Calming
RutaVaLa
Sacred Mountain
Stress Away Roll-on
Tranquil Roll-on

SUPPLEMENTS:

ImmuPro
Multigreens
NingXia Red
Sleepessence

sad, grouchy, and depressed. Over time you may find you are not only unable to sleep but experience a dull ache in your lower back. Try drinking an ounce of **NingXia Red** with 2 **Multigreen** capsules instead of caffeine and sugar in the morning. Applying **Nutmeg** and **Sandalwood** to the lower back can help support your adrenals.

A ruffled mind makes a restless pillow.

—Charlotte Brontë—

Suggested Reading

Complete Guide to Natural Sleep by Dian Dincin Buchman (Jun 1, 1997)

Releasing Emotional Patterns with Essential Oils, NEW - Updated Edition for 2011 by Dr. Carolyn L. Mein (Paperback, 2011)

Healing with Aromatherapy by Marlene Ericksen (2003)

Sore Throat

There are many reasons why sore throats arise. Whether it's post nasal drip from allergies, or swelling from a virus or an infection, that familiar pain is one that we all want to get rid of quickly.

Tip: Zinc has been shown to be a very effective sore throat fighter. Our favorite supplements for zinc are: *SuperCal*, *Super C*, & *True Source*.

Our Approach:

Apply: One to two drops of *Lemon*, *Lavender*, and/or *Thieves* (diluted) to the outside of the throat. Still have pain? Add 1-3 drops of diluted *PanAway* or *Clove* on top of the other oils.

Try: Gargling with *Thieves Mouthwash* and sucking on *Thieves Lozenges* periodically during the day. Spray *Thieves Spray* in the mouth and back of the throat. Drink an oz. of *NingXia Red* with 2 drops each of **Lemon** & *Frankincense* 2-3 times a day. Take 1-2 *ImmuPro* tablets and a *Life 5* capsule at night.

Diffuse: *Ecualyptus Blue* and/or *Melrose* during the day and *Lavender* at night.

Did you know?

Sore throats are often the first sign of an illness. If you ignore your sore throat you will often be on a longer path to wellness.

Providing a humidifier, or cool mist diffuser (with essential oils) in your child's bedroom is also helpful in reducing the dry air which can aggravate any sore throat. — Dr. Mary Ann LoFrumento

Gargling is an excellent way to deal with a sore throat. Try adding essential oils to salt & water and gargling with this mixture for as long as you can. — Andrew Weil, MD.

Remember to order everything needed for the cold & flu seasons before they begin: fall, winter, and summer. Be sure to order from the YL90 Plan brochure, *Cold-n-Flu Fighters*, before each season.

We like to diffuse year round to keep germs and toxins at bay. Some oils are more costly than others, so keep the more expensive oils for applying and the less expensive oils for diffusing. Inexpensive Lemon oil is great for diffusing and great for a sore throat.

Dear Carrie & Elena,

Whenever my throat gets sore, I spray the Thieves Spray in my mouth, and it helps right away. Recently when I didn't have the spray with me, I tried a drop of peppermint, and that too brought immediate relief. It gave me the idea that I may want to use them together from now on! Now I find that even when I don't have a sore throat, it helps to keep my breath fresh.

—Fred D., NJ

A good listener is not someone with nothing to say. A good listener is a talker with a sore throat.

—Katherine Elizabeth Whitehorn—

| Suggested Reading | *Better Health through Natural Healing* by Dr. Ross Trattler, ND, DO and Dr. Adrian Jones, ND. (Paperback, 2001)

New Guide to Remedies by Parragon Publishing Group. (Hardcover, 2005) | *Aromatherapy: A Complete Guide to the Healing Art* by Kathi Keville & Mindy Green (Paperback)

Growing Up Green: Baby and Child Care by Deirdre Imus (Paperback, April 5, 2008) |

Sports Performance

Most people start an exercise program knowing what equipment to use and even how to dress; but how often do we consider what additional nutrition we may need? Here is a place to start...

Our Approach:

Apply: *OrthoSport* massage oil to the entire body after bathing to prevent injury. Our muscles work in groups and we tend to compensate on one side when the other is weakened.

Try: A *Power Meal* or *Pure Protein Complete* shake to give your body extra nutrition. Taking a shot of **NingXia Red** and 2-3 **Multigreen** capsules 2-3 times a day may help to boost your energy level and endurance.

Diffuse: *Peppermint* may help to increase mental acuity and athletic performance.

Did you know?

Dehydroepiandrosterone (DHEA) is a hormone that is made naturally by the adrenal glands. It is used to help make the sex hormones testosterone and estrogen, and is found in **PD 80/20, UltraYoung, EndoGize, & Cortistop**

DHEA is used for osteoporosis prevention, support of the adrenal glands, and for immune support. It may also improve sexual function in men and women and help relieve depression. Athletes use DHEA because they believe that DHEA will suppress cortisol, the stress hormone. —Cathy Wong, *Alternative Medicine Guide*

Tip: Recent studies support that physical performance is seasonal. When Vitamin D levels peak due to sun exposure, physical performance peaks as well. Get out side and get fit! — Dr. Joseph Mercola

We've all heard the expression, "no pain, no gain." Pain is our body's way of telling us we are working hard, but it is also our body's signal to either slow down or work smarter. Use healthy supplementation to support stress on our body and be proactive with the right essential oils to make all the difference when dealing with injury.

Follow our 90-day plan in the YL90 Plan brochure, *Live Pain Free,* and stay on track

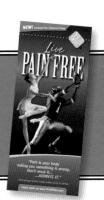

Dear Carrie & Elena,

While away on a weekend trip, I "over exercised" and injured my neck and shoulder muscles. My range of motion was seriously decreased and I was in a panic about having to drive home in the car for 6 hours the next day. Fortunately, one of my travel companions had a supply of BLM and Sulfurzyme. One capsule of each, every hour got me home and I was even able to drive comfortably!

—Lisa S., NJ

Games lubricate the body and the mind.

—Benjamin Franklin—

Suggested Reading	Aroma Yoga by Tracy Griffiths (2010)	The Eat-Clean Diet Workout: Quick Routines for
	DHEA: The Youth and Health Hormone by C. Norman Shealy, M.D., Ph.D. (Paperback, Jan. 1, 1999)	Your Best Body Ever (with DVD) by Tosca Reno (Paperback, Dec. 3, 2007)
	A New Route to Robust Health By D. Gary Young, N.D., (Paperback, 2000)	

Stress Relief & Relaxation

Daily relaxation is a necessity for good health and to help balance the physical & emotional stresses of life. Stress compounds over time and can do cumulative damage. The solution is a combination of good nutrition, exercise, & sleep.

· · · · · · ·

Tip: *Idaho Balsam Fir* can help to reduce cortisol levels (stress hormones). Apply or diffuse this oil in the morning before you face the world. Take some time to pray or meditate while diffusing. Take a walk and breathe...deeply.

· · · · · · ·

Our Approach:

Apply: *Stress Away Roll-on* to your pulse points. Carry this with you and reapply as necessary. Alternate with **Valor**, **Lavender**, and **Peace & Calming**. Apply **Nutmeg** to your lower back to support your adrenals. After an evening shower or bath, apply **Relaxation Massage Oil** to your body.

Try: One oz. of **NingXia Red** and 2 **Multigreen** capsules during the day to keep your daytime energy up, so that you can sleep more restfully at night. Twenty minutes before bed, take 1-2 **ImmuPro** tablets or **Sleepessence** capsules to promote a full night's sleep. You can also put a drop of **Valerian** under your tongue. A good night's sleep will bring down your stress levels the next day.

Diffuse: Your favorite calming oil. We like **Lavender**, **Peace & Calming**, **Stress Away Roll-on**, **Bergamot**, or **Sacred Mountain**.

Did you know?

Busy people often feel anxious, depressed, or exhausted. They also may have short fuses, gain weight easily, or have weak immune systems. These symptoms can often be attributed to one thing: adrenal fatigue. The stress of living in overdrive on a daily basis can burn you out.

Jump start your stress reduction program with a Raindrop Treatment. Look online for the practitioner nearest you or get a Raindrop Kit from Young Living and have a friend or family member follow the enclosed instructional DVD.

Afterwards, follow our nutritional program in the YL90 Plan brochure, *Who Needs a Raindrop? Everybody!* to continue on a healthy path to stress reduction and revitalization.

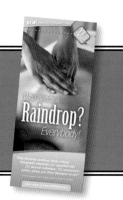

Dear Carrie & Elena,

Some days are naturally more stressful than others, and on those days I keep my Stress Away Roll-On right beside me on my desk. I lather it on, and it always gives me great relief. God definitely provided for every ailment under the sun!

—Don S., NJ

SINGLES:

Bergamot
Idaho Balsam Fir
Lavender
Nutmeg
Valerian

OIL BLENDS:

Peace & Calming
Sacred Mountain
Stress Away Roll-on
Valor

SUPPLEMENTS:

ImmuPro
Multigreens
NingXia Red
Sleepessence

PERSONAL CARE:

Relaxation
    Massage Oil

A crust eaten in peace
is better than a banquet
eaten in anxiety.

—Aesop—

| Suggested Reading | A More Excellent Way - Be In Health by Henry Wright (2005) | Feelings Buried Alive Never Die by Karol Kuhn Truman (Aug 1, 1991) | Molecules Of Emotion: The Science Behind Mind-Body Medicine by Candace B. Pert (Feb 17, 1999) |

Virus

Viruses, according to the Mayo Clinic are "capsules", smaller than cells, that contain genetic material. To reproduce, viruses invade cells of the body, hijacking the machinery that makes cells work. Host cells are eventually destroyed during this process. Viruses are responsible for everything from AIDS to the common cold, including Ebola Virus, hemorrhagic fever, genital herpes, influenza, measles, smallpox, herpes, molluscum, chicken pox, & shingles.

Our Approach:

Apply: Oils often! A drop or two of **Melaleuca Alternifolia**, **Melissa**, **Rosemary**, **Thieves**, **Oregano**, **Sandalwood**, or **Thyme** to the bottom of the feet and along the spine (diluted).

Try: One to two oz. of **NingXia Red**, an **Inner Defense** capsule, & a **Life 5** capsule (right before bed) during the day; and **ImmuPro** tablets or **Sleepessence** capsules at night (20 minutes before you want to retire). You can also put a drop of **Melissa** under your tongue.

Diffuse: A good germ-fighting oil. Our favorites are **Thieves**, **Lemon**, **Purification**, **RC**, and **Ecualyptus Blue**.

Did you know?

Coconut oil is highly antiviral. Bruce Fife, C.N., N.D. and author of *The Coconut Oil Miracle* shares, "Laboratory tests have shown that the MCFAs (medium chain fatty acids) found in coconut oil are effective in destroying viruses that cause influenza, measles, herpes, mononucleosis hepatitis C, and AIDS; bacteria that can cause stomach ulcers, throat infections, pneumonia, sinusitis, urinary tract infections, meningitis, gonorrhea, and toxic shock syndrome; fungi and yeast that lead to ringworm, candida, and thrush; and parasites that can cause intestinal infections such as giardiasis."

Did you know that using essential oils with whole food supplements is more effective than taking each one alone? Just like a good sauce has many ingredients, good health comes from many sources.

Follow our 90-day plan to good health and cold and flu prevention in the YL90 Plan brochure, *Cold-n-Flu Fighters*, and create a comprehensive plan for your health that works.

Dear Carrie & Elena,

Di-Gize works wonders! Whenever I feel nauseous or have diarrhea, I rub Di-Gize on my stomach every couple of hours. It gets rid of the nausea and if it is not a bad bug I'm usually better within 24 hours or less.

—Dalton H., WI

Shopping List

SINGLES:

Eucalyptus Blue
Lemon
Melaleuca Alternifolia
Melissa
Oregano
Rosemary
Sandalwood
Thyme

OIL BLENDS:

Di-Gize
Purification
RC
Thieves

SUPPLEMENTS:

Balance Complete
ImmuPro
Inner Defense
Life 5
NingXia Red
Sleepessence

PERSONAL CARE:

Thieves Cleaner
Thieves Hand Purifier
Thieves Spray

Look for natural supplement products with coconut oil, our favorites are: **Balance Complete**, **Inner Defense**, and **ImmuPro**.

. . . .

Tip: If you don't have **Thieves** in your house, now is the time to start. Rob the virus of its strength. Diffuse **Thieves Oil Blend**, clean with **Thieves Cleaner**, spray **Thieves Spray** on phones, light switches, & door knobs, and use **Thieves Hand Purifier** on hands.

. . . .

"I pictured myself as a virus or a cancer cell and tried to sense what it would be like."

—Jonas Salk—

| **Suggested Reading** | *The Coconut Oil Miracle* (Previously published as *The Healing Miracle of Coconut Oil*) by Bruce Fife and Jon J. Kabara (Sep 9, 2004) | *What to do When Antibiotics Don't Work! How to Stay Healthy and Alive When Infections Strike* by Dirk Van Gils (Paperback, 2002) | *Aromatherapy: An A-Z* by Patricia Davis (2000) |

Vision

Vision problems can include changes in vision, glaucoma, cataracts, or even macular degeneration. The foods we eat, how we take care of our eyes, and the amount of sleep we get all factor into eye health.

....

Tip: The compounds in *Frankincense*, including boswellic acid, are very healing to the eyes. Their anti-inflammatory powers and ancient historical uses demonstrate their effective applications in eye health.
—Dr. Ray Sahelian, MD

....

Our Approach:

Apply: One to two drops of *Frankincense*, diluted, around the eyes with *Boswellia Wrinkle Cream* on top.

Try: One to two oz. of *NingXia Red*, 3 *OmegaGize* capsules, & a *Longevity* capsule 1-2 times daily.

Diffuse: *Peace & Calming* or *Lavender* to help you sleep at night. A good night's rest is very important for eye health.

Did you know?

One of the keys to good vision health is carotenoids? Carotenoids are natural pigments which are synthesized by plants and are responsible for the bright colors of various fruits and vegetables. Young Living's *Power Meal*, *Balance Complete*, and *NingXia Red* are full of carotenoids--replace one meal a day or add as a snack. Potent antioxidants, such as anthocyanin, flavanoids, and carotenoids can also be found in blueberries. Studies have shown that the anthocyanins in blueberries support healthy neurological function and aid in normal eye health.

Purchasing therapeutic-grade products is critical. This grade sets the essential oil apart from other essential oils because, from planting to harvesting to marketing, the process is carefully monitored. By following the YL90 Plan's guide to using your oils properly in our *Essential Oil Basics* brochure, you will get the most from your products.

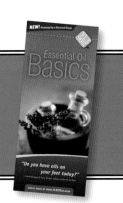

Dear Carrie & Elena,

For the past 24 years, every eye doctor visit meant a new prescription for me. My eyesight has slowly gotten worse over the course of my life. After drinking NingXia Red over the course of one year, my most recent eye doctors visit proved no change in my eyesight! No better, but no worse!

—Erin G., Lil Shop of Oils, LLC, OH

Increasing the amount of lutein, zeaxanthin, and carotenoids can help improve your fight against macular degeneration. These antioxidants are found in **Sulfurzyme**, **NingXia Red**, **Balance Complete**, **Power Meal**, **True Source**, and **MightyVites**.

"Antioxidants have been shown to significantly reduce the occurrence of chronic diseases that do significant and progressive damage to the body over time. Prevent this breakdown with the right nutrition." —*www.mdsupport.org*

"God, grant me the senility to forget the people I never liked anyway, the good fortune to run into the ones I do, and the eyesight to tell the difference."

—Anonymous—

Suggested Reading

Discovery of the Ultimate Superfood: How the Ningxia Wolfberry And 4 Other Foods Help Combat Heart Disease, Cancer, Chronic Fatigue, Depression, Diabetes And More by Gary Young, Marc Schreuder and Ronald, Ph.D. Lawrence (Paperback, July 30, 2005)

Better Health Through Natural Healing: How to Get Well Without Drugs or Surgery by Ross Trattler and Adrian Jones (Paperback, Aug. 2004)

Weight Management

Culture, age, sex, diet, sleep, stress, exercise, and medications all factor into to our ability to manage an ideal weight. Everyone can have the weight that they desire with the right formula.

· · · · · · ·

Tip: Hungry? Drink a glass of water with a few drops of citrus oil or a cup of Slique Tea either hot or cold. Most of us are not really hungry, we are thirsty. Fill the void with hydration instead of empty calories. Need something to crunch on? Try a water-rich whole-food like cucumbers or watermelon.

· · · · · · ·

Our Approach:

Apply: Wear **Black Pepper** and your favorite citrus oil: **Grapefruit, Orange, Lemon, Tangerine,** or **Bergamot** to help reduce cravings and as your favorite weight loss cologne. **Dill** worn on the wrists also works as an effective craving reducer.

Try: Try a capsule with 3 drops each of: **Grapefruit, Tangerine, Spearmint, Lemon,** and **Ocotea.** A few drops of Slique Essence in warm or cold drinks to help reduce the desire for sugary beverages.

Diffuse: **Citrus Fresh,** we find this blend helps to remove the desire to eat.

Dear Carrie & Elena,

When I find myself up a few pounds, there's no better jump start to weight loss than the 5-Day Cleanse. I find that this cleanse is very gentle, yet effective in helping the body release excess pounds. I find it to be the perfect jump start to a weight loss program, since I always see fast results. I drink citrus oils in my water every day, which helps me release the toxins. I also like taking Comfortone when I am doing the 5-Day Cleanse, as I find that really gets the colon moving. Releasing the toxins first with a cleanse is a great way to start a weight management program.

—Leanne G., NJ

Many people understand the need to cut calories and exercise more. The key to losing fat is incorporating fat burning foods, supplements, and essential oils into our daily routine. The list on the next page details the information on the oils and supplements listed in the YL90 Plan brochure, *Fat Loss that Works*, which provides a chart of these great fat burners. Pick at least one every time you eat and you will see the pounds start to melt away and the lean you show through!

> *In eating, a third of the stomach should be filled with food, a third with drink and the rest left empty.*
>
> —Talmud—

Top Oils and Supplements for Weight Management

Essential Oils may:

Black Pepper: reduce hunger, create a feeling of fullness, & reduce fat stores

Citrus Fresh: increase metabolism, drain the lymphatic system, & curb cravings

Cypress: reduce cellulite, increase detoxification, and improve circulation

Dill: support the pancreas and normalize insulin levels

Ginger: burn more calories and release fat from fat stores

Grapefruit: breakdown fats

Lemon: neutralize acids to help release toxins from fat cells

Ocotea: balance blood sugar

Orange: increase metabolism and aid digestion

Slique Essence: ingredients help to control hunger and act as an all-natural sweetener

Tangerine: remove toxins from fat cells and improve digestion

Supplements may:

Balance Complete: increase appetite satisfaction and balance blood sugar

Blue Agave: give you the sweet taste you are looking for in a healthier way

Digest & Cleanse: improve digestion and aid in cleansing

Essentialzymes-4: improve digestion and eliminate toxins from the body

Life 5: improve digestion and increase the number of calories burned

Longevity: clean toxins and burn fat

Multigreens: increase metabolism and burn fat

NingXia Red: increase energy and reduce cravings

OmegaGize : increase the number of calories burned in a day

Slique Tea: helps reduce appetite and provides a natural energy boost

True Source: increase energy and improve nutrition

Shopping List

SINGLES:

Black Pepper
Cypress
Dill
Ginger
Grapefruit
Lemon
Ocotea
Orange
Peppermint
Tangerine

OIL BLENDS:

Slique Essence
Citrus Fresh

SUPPLEMENTS:

Balance Complete
Blue Agave
Comfortone
Digest & Cleanse
Essentialzymes-4
5-Day Cleanse
Life 5
Longevity
Multigreens
NingXia Red
OmegaGize
Slique Tea
True Source

Suggested Reading

The Eat-Clean Diet: Fast Fat-Loss that lasts Forever! by Tosca Reno (Jan 8, 2007)

Fast Food Nation: The Dark Side of the All-American Meal by Eric Schlosser (Paperback, July 5, 2005)

Milk - The Deadly Poison by Robert Cohen and Brian Vigorita (Hardcover, Nov. 1, 1997)

Eat to Live: The Amazing Nutrient-Rich Program for Fast and Sustained Weight Loss, Revised Edition by Joel Fuhrman (Jan 5, 2011)

Nutritarian Handbook by Joel and M.D. Fuhrman (Aug 26, 2010)

Women's Health

Women face unique health challenges from PMS to menopause, weight changes, childbirth, bone loss, headaches, memory, and more. So much about being a woman is multitasking. Keeping stress down and energy high is a winning ticket to any woman's health.

. . . .

Tip: Lowering cortisol may not only improve how you feel but how you look. Improve your skin, hair, and appearance by reducing or eliminating coffee and other sources of caffeine; begin drinking water with essential oils. Supercharge your day with a shot of **NingXia Red**.

. . . .

Our Approach:

Apply: One to two drops of **Believe**, **En-R-Gee**, or **Gratitude** on your pulse points. A few drops of **Progessence Plus** to belly or thighs can help with low progesterone levels; **Sclaressence** to ankles for low estrogen levels; & **M-Grain** *or* **Basil** to temples for migraines.

Try: One **PD 80/20** capsule for overall hormone support, **True Source** vitamins or **Master Formula Hers** vitamins for better nutrition, and 2 **Cortistop** capsules to support balanced cortisol levels.

Diffuse: **Idaho Balsam Fir**, **Believe**, or **Cedarwood**, all oils and blends that that come from trees can very supportive of a woman's mind, body, and soul.

Did you know?

The biggest challenge to a woman's health is the queen of stress hormones: cortisol. A stress-filled life, lack of sleep, age, environmental and nutritional stresses, lack of exercise, and caffeine drive cortisol to dangerous levels. Cortisol inhibits the growth of beneficial microflora in the intestines. These essential bacteria support the immune system, create B vitamins, and increase the absorption of minerals like calcium, iron, and magnesium. A decrease in their population results in more colds, sore throats, headaches, diarrhea, upset stomachs and the overgrowth of harmful bacteria and fungus like candida.

Hormones can be a tricky business. Symptons like: weight gain, headaches, change in body structure, hair loss, bone loss, lack of energy, and more are often caused by hormone imbalance.

Start using the YL90 Core Program for Women in the YL90 Plan brochure, *Healthy Woman: Hormone Rescue Guide,* and support your hormones from the inside out.

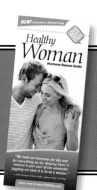

Dear Carrie & Elena,

I can't say enough about Progessence Plus. I was a widow who had closed herself off emotionally and Progessence Plus opened me up to feeling like a woman again. It also has helped me to lose weight and have a more positive attitude. Using a few drops each day has changed my life immeasurably.

—Lillian B. NJ

SINGLES:
  Basil
  Cedarwood
  Idaho Balsam Fir

OIL BLENDS:
  Believe
  En-R-Gee
  Gratitude
  M-Grain
  Sclaressence

SUPPLEMENTS:
  Cortistop
  Master Formula Hers
  NingXia Red
  PD 80/20
  True Source

PERSONAL CARE:
  Progessence Plus

Moodiness, anxiety, and depression & headaches are all consequences of elevated cortisol's long-term effects on seratonin and dopamine production and may even cause brain cells to actually shrink!

One is not born a woman, one becomes one.

—Simone de Beauvoir—

Suggested Reading	*Progesterone: the Ultimate Woman's Feel-Good Hormone* by Dan Purser, MD (Booklet, 2010)	*Women's Bodies, Women's Wisdom* by Christiane Northrup, M.D. (Paperback, June 1, 2010).	*Mother-Daughter Wisdom: Understanding the Crucial Link Between Mothers, Daughters, and Health* by Christiane Northrup (Mar 28, 2006)

Glossary of Blends & Supplements

Blends

Abundance – Attract prosperity; *Contains: orange, clove, cinnamon bark,* frankincense, ginger, spruce, patchouli, myrrh

Aroma Life – Promote heart vitality; Contains: cypress, helichrysum, ylang ylang marjoram

Aroma Siez – Relax tight muscles and ligaments; Contains: basil, lavender, cypress, marjoram, peppermint

Believe – Encourages feelings of strength and faith; Contains: balsam fir, rosewood, frankincense

Brain Power – Give your brain a boost, clarify thought and develop greater focus; Contains: sandalwood, Melissa, helichrysum, cedarwood, blue cypress, frankincense, lavender

Breathe Again – Support respiratory health; Contains: coconut oil, eucalyptus staigeriana, eucalyptus globulus, laurus nobilis, rose hip fruit oil, peppermint, eucalyptus radiata, copaiba, myrtle, blue cypress oil, eucalyptus blue

Citrus Fresh – Stimulate mental activity, boost creativity; Contains: orange, grapefruit, mandarin, tangerine, lemon, spearmint

Clarity – Restore mental alertness; Contains: basil, rosewood, roman chamomile, cardamom, geranium, bergamot, rosemary, lemon, ylang ylang peppermint, jasmine, palmarosa

Deep Relief – Provides support for head and muscle tension Contains: peppermint, balsam fir, clove, vetiver, wintergreen, lemon, helichrysum, copaiba, coconut oil.

Di-Gize – Promote healthy digestion and soothe stomach discomforts; Contains: tarragon, juniper, anise, ginger, fennel, patchouli, peppermint, lemongrass

En-R-Gee – Uplift and energize mind and body; Contains: rosemary, nutmeg, pepper, juniper, balsam fir, lemongrass, clove

Gentle Baby – Helps calm emotions for mothers and children; Contains: geranium, jasmine, ylang ylang, roman chamomile, rose, lemon, bergamot, lavender, palmarosa

GLF – Gallbladder & Liver Flush, helps eliminate the negative effects of toxins in the body; Contains: grapefruit, ledum, helichrysum, hyssop, celery, spearmint

Gratitude – Supports emotional and spiritual progress; Contains: balsam fir, rosewood, galbanum, frankincense, myrrh, ylang ylang

Harmony – Can help bring harmonic balance to the energy centers (chakras) of the body; Contains: geranium, angelica, bergamot, lavender, spruce, ylang ylang, sandalwood, hyssop, palmarosa, rosewood, Spanish sage, rose, frankincense, jasmine, lemon, orange, Roman chamomile

Immupower – Formulated to support the body's natural immune system when applied to the Vitaflex points on the hands and feet; Contains: hyssop, ravensara, clove, mountain savory, frankincense, cumin, cistus, oregano, Idaho tansy

Inspiration – Enhance spirituality and meditation, can be used before starting work each day; Contains: cedarwood, myrtle, mugwort, spruce, sandalwood, rosewood, frankincense

Joy – Can help bring happiness to the heart; Contains: bergamot, lemon, palmarosa, ylang ylang, mandarin, rose, geranium, jasmine, rosewood, roman chamomile

Juva Cleanse – Supports healthy liver function; Contains: helichrysum, ledum

Live With Passion – Helps revive enthusiasm for life and love; Contains: clary sage, ginger, sandalwood, angelica, cedarwood, helichrysum, jasmine, melissa, neroli, patchouli

Melrose – Helps combat minor skin irritations and infection; Contains: rosemary, clove, melaleuca alternifolia, niaouli

M-Grain – soothes head and muscle tension; Contains: basil, lavender, roman chamomile, marjoram, peppermint, helichrysum

Mister – Helps men to balance emotions during stressful times; Contains: sage, lavender, peppermint, fennel, myrtle, blue yarrow

PanAway – Aids the body's natural response to pain & injury. Minimizes bruising, relieves muscle tension; Contains: wintergreen, clove, helichrysum, peppermint

Peace & Calming – Encourages deep relaxation to promote a peaceful night's sleep; Contains: tangerine, ylangylang, blue tansy, orange, patchouli

Purification – Deodorizes and neutralizes the air, contains citronella to deter insects & soothe minor bites;
Contains: lemongrass, rosemary, melaleuca, myrtle, citronella

Raven – Deeply soothing to the chest and throat when applied topically;
Contains: ravensara, wintergreen, eucalyptus radiata, lemon, peppermint

RC – Deeply soothing to the chest and throat when applied topically;
Contains: eucalyptus globulus, myrtle, spruce, eucalyptus radiata, eucalyptus citriodora, peppermint, pine, lavender, marjoram, cypress

Relieve it – Soothes muscle and joint discomfort
Contains: spruce, black pepper, peppermint

RutaVaLa – Helps relieve stress, soothes tension and promotes relaxation of mind and body
Contains: Lavender, valerian, ruta graveolens

Sacred Mountain – Promotes feelings of strength, grounding and protection;
Contains: spruce, balsam fir, ylangylang, cedarwood

Sclaressence – helps support women's hormonal health;
Contains: clary sage, fennel, sage, lavender, peppermint

Sensation – Encourage feelings of love and affection;
Contains: rosewood, ylangylang, jasmine

Slique Essence - Supports healthy weight-management goals;
Contains: grapefruit, tangerine, lemon, spearmint, and ocotea essential oils with stevia extract

Stress Away – Help relieve daily stress, encourage relaxation,
Contains: vanilla, lime, copaiba

Surrender – Cast off feelings that may be limiting your potential;
Contains: lavender, spruce, mountain savory, lemon, angelica, roman chamomile, german chamomile

Thieves – Helps kill dangerous airborne bacteria or can be applied to the body for immune support;
Contains: clove, cinnamon bark, rosemary, lemon, eucalyptus radiata

Tranquil – Help decrease anxiety;
Contains: lavender, cedarwood, roman chamomile, coconut oil

V-6 Mixing Oil – a blend of fatty vegetable oils, can be used to dilute essential oils on sensitive skin
Contains: coconut oil, sesame seed oil, grape seed oil, sweet almond oil, wheat germ oil, sunflower seed oil, olive fruit oil

Valor – Helps promote feelings of courage ad security; helps with the alignment of the body;
Contains: spruce, blue tansy, rosewood, frankincense

White Angelica – Can be used to guard against negative energy;
Contains: bergamot, rosewood, Melissa, geranium, ylangylang, rose, myrrh, spruce, sandalwood, hyssop

Supplements

Alkalime: Essential oils and minerals in a powder to help balance the body's pH

Balance Complete: Essential Oil infused superfood-meal replacement shake

BLM: To support bones, ligaments, joints, and muscles with the oils of Idaho Balsam Fir, clove & natural ingredients such as Type II Collagen, MSM, & glucosamine sulphate.

Blue Agave: Organic nectar from Agave Tequilana; a safe alternative to sugar or artificial sweeteners.

Cleansing Trio: ICP, Comfortone, & Essentialzyme are enhanced with minerals, enzymes, amino acids, fiber, and essential oils to help eliminate waste in the body and support overall health

Comfortone: Combines fiber, minerals, herbs, and the essential oils ginger and peppermint to support digestion

Cortistop: Helps support the female glandular system and balance cortisol with frankincense, peppermint, & fennel

Digest & Cleanse: Helps support natural digestion with ginger, lemon, fennel, and peppermint

Core Supplements: Provides daily foundational nutrition in easy to use am, noon, and pm packets. Includes: True Source, OmegaGize , Longevity, and Life 5

Endogize: Support a healthy endocrine system with natural herbs and clary sage and myrrh essential oils

Essentialzyme: Multi-enzyme complex to promote good digestion with peppermint and fennel

5-Day Nutritive Cleanse: Promotes gentle and effective cleansing with NingXia Red, Balance Complete, and Digest & Cleanse

ICP: Supports colon health with a mix of soluble and insoluble fibers, enzymes, and lemongrass essential oil

ImmuPro: Combines NingXia wolfberries, orange essential oil, calcium, zinc, miatake, & reishi mushrooms

Inner Defense: Immproves the body's defenses with oregano and Thieves oil

Life 5: High-potency probiotic that supports core intestinal health

Longevity: Softgels with frankincense, clove, thyme, and orange

Master Formula Hers: To support the nutritional needs of woman with vitamins, minerals, antioxidants, and other nutrients

Master Formula His: To support the nutritional needs of men with vitamins, minerals, antioxidants, and other nutrients

MegaCal: Calcium and mineral powder to support vascular and bone health

Mineral Essence: Liquid mineral enhanced with lemon and cinnamon bark oils

Multigreens: A blend of chlorophyll, rich botanicals, choline, and amino acids to boost vitality and reduce stress

NingXia Red: A combination of: whole NingXia wolfberries, blueberries, raspberries and red grapes with lemon and orange essential oils. A powerful antioxidant-rich liquid, fruit puree containing fiber, protein and a variety of vitamins and minerals

OmegaGize: A clinically-proven dose of omega-3 fatty acids with blue chamomile, lemongrass, and clove essential oils

PD 80/20: Formulated to replenish the body's pregnenolone and DHEA

Power Meal: Vegetarian, rice-based meal replacement shake rich in calcium, antioxidants, and amino acids and enhanced with lemon, grapefruit essential oils

Prostate Health: Fast-acting, vegetable-based herbal product formulated with saw-palmetto for prostate health

Pure Protein Complete: Protein shake with 20 grams of protein from whey and orange essential oil, vitamins, and minerals

Slique Tea: Helps support individual weight goals;
Contains: oolong tea, inulin, ocotea leaf, cacao powder, vanilla essential oil, frankincense powder and natural stevia extract

Sleepessence: Lavender, Vetivier, valerian with melatonin for a great night's sleep

Sulfurzyme: Natural form of MSM, a dietary sulfur to support normal metabolism and circulation

Super B: A blend of 8 essential B vitamins

Super C: Vitamin C combined with minerals, bioflavonoids, and orange & lemon essential oils

Super Cal: Combines calcium, magnesium, potassium and zinc with wintergreen and lemongrass essential oils

Thyromin: A blend of bovine glandular extracts, herbs, and amino acids, minerals, myrrh and spearmint essential oils to support the thyroid

True Source: Whole-food based multivitamin

Index

YL90 Plan *(Your Life in 90 Days)*

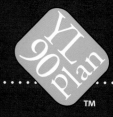

Collect all of these smart, helpful, time-saving and beautiful brochures by best-selling authors Carrie Donegan & Elena Yordán.

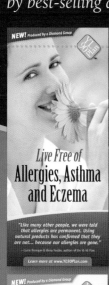

NEW! Produced by a Diamond Group

Live Free of
**Allergies, Asthma
and Eczema**

"Like many other people, we were told that allergies are permanent. Using natural products has confirmed that they are not... because our allergies are gone."
—Carrie Donegan & Elena Yordán, authors of the YL-90 Plan

Learn more at www.YL90Plan.com

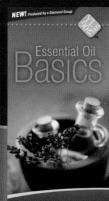

NEW! Produced by a Diamond Group

Essential Oil
Basics

*"Do you have oils on
your feet today?"*
—Carrie Donegan & Elena Yordán, authors of the YL-90 Plan

Learn more at www.YL90Plan.com

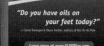

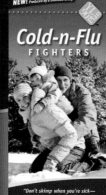

NEW! Produced by a Diamond Group

**Cold-n-Flu
FIGHTERS**

"Don't skimp when you're sick—more is more, don't drip, pour! Applications can be repeated multiple times throughout the day."
—Carrie Donegan & Elena Yordán, authors of the YL-90 Plan

Learn more at www.YL90Plan.com

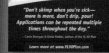

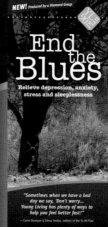

NEW! Produced by a Diamond Group

**End
the
Blues**
Relieve depression, anxiety,
stress and sleeplessness

"Sometimes when we have a bad day we say, 'Don't worry...' Young Living has plenty of ways to help you feel better fast!"
—Carrie Donegan & Elena Yordán, authors of the YL-90 Plan

Learn more at www.YL90Plan.com

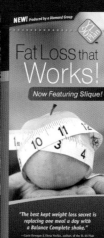

NEW! Produced by a Diamond Group

Fat Loss that
Works!
Now Featuring Slique!

"The best kept weight loss secret is replacing one meal a day with a Balance Complete shake."
—Carrie Donegan & Elena Yordán, authors of the YL-90 Plan

Learn more at www.YL90Plan.com

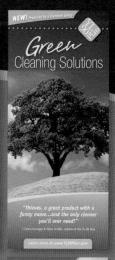

NEW! Produced by a Diamond Group

Green
Cleaning Solutions

"Thieves, a great product with a funny name...and the only cleaner you'll ever need!"
—Carrie Donegan & Elena Yordán, authors of the YL-90 Plan

Learn more at www.YL90Plan.com

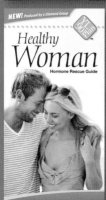

NEW! Produced by a Diamond Group

Healthy
Woman
Hormone Rescue Guide

"We need our hormones for life and for everything we do. Keeping them in balance is just part of the wonderful juggling act that it is to be a women."
—Carrie Donegan & Elena Yordán, authors of the YL-90 Plan

Learn more at www.YL90Plan.com

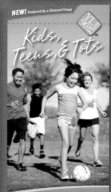

NEW! Produced by a Diamond Group

*Kids,
Teens, & Tots*

"We met because we were two moms on a mission to remove toxins from our kid's lives. Natural is best and safest for our families."
—Carrie Donegan & Elena Yordán, authors of the YL-90 Plan

Learn more at www.YL90Plan.com

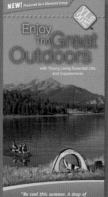

NEW! Produced by a Diamond Group

Enjoy
The **Great**
Outdoors
with Young Living Essential Oils
and Supplements

"Be cool this summer. A drop of peppermint on the back of the neck is a sure-fire way to cool down —no air conditioning needed!"
—Carrie Donegan & Elena Yordán, authors of the YL-90 Plan

Learn more at www.YL90Plan.com

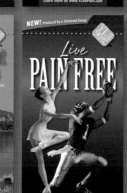

Live
PAIN FREE

"Pain is your body telling you something is wrong. Don't mask it... ...ADDRESS IT."
—Carrie Donegan & Elena Yordán, authors of the YL-90 Plan

Learn more at www.YL90Plan.com

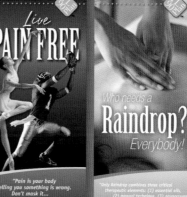

NEW! Produced by a Diamond Group

Who needs a
Raindrop?
Everybody!

"Only Raindrop combines three critical therapeutic elements: (1) essential oils, (2) manual technique, (3) acupressure points; giving you three therapies in one"
—Carrie Donegan & Elena Yordán, authors of the YL-90 Plan

Learn more at www.YL90Plan.com

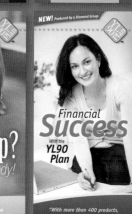

NEW! Produced by a Diamond Group

Financial
Success
With the
**YL90
Plan**

"With more than 400 products, it's hard to know how to start. The YL90 Plan gets you going fast!"
—Carrie Donegan & Elena Yordán, authors of the YL-90 Plan

Learn more at www.YL90Plan.com

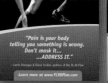

Maximize your sharing power without spending a lot!

Now also available in Spanish or German!

Follow us online:

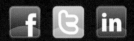

Join in the fun at
facebook.com/YL90Plan *&*
facebook.com/Essential Oils 101

Follow the YL90 Plan
@yl90plan

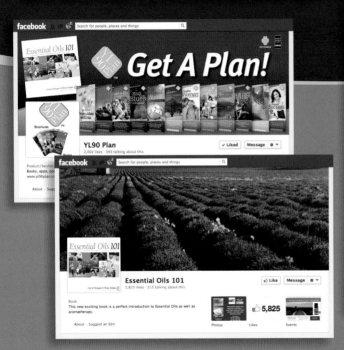

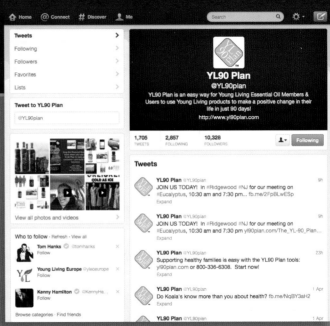

Join the YL90 Plan Facebook page to interact and communicate with other essential oils users just like you! Frequent posts, contests, videos, and information all for free. This is a friendly community of users created just for you.

Swap:
- Tips
- Information
- Studies
- New Ideas
- Encouragement
- Experiences

Get up-to-the-minute insights from the YL90 Plan as we tweet about oils, travels, events, books, magazines, brochures and more!

Be the first to know -
follow the YL90 Plan on Twitter!

Buy the App: *(Available for both Android and Apple)*

Introducing the YL90 App! Your quick essential reference to essential oils and YL90 plans.

What is a YL90 plan? A YL90 plan is a 90-day plan to help you use essential oils and aromatherapy to bring out the best in you. In the app are plans to help with everything from relieving allergies to fighting depression!

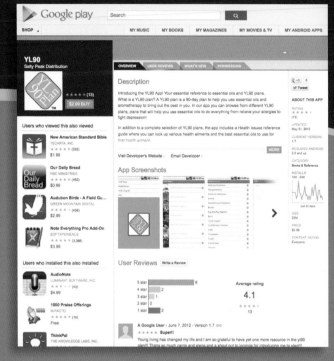

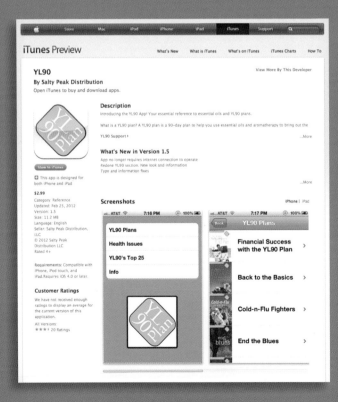

In addition to a complete selection of YL90 plans, the app includes a Health Issues reference guide where you can look up various health concerns and helpful essential oils.

The app also includes top recomended products; a reference guide you can use to look up individual oils & products and their application.

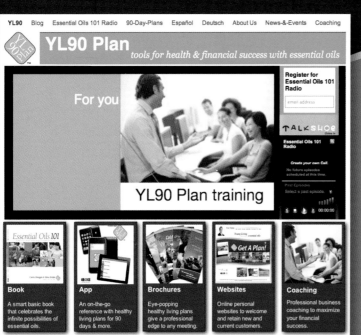
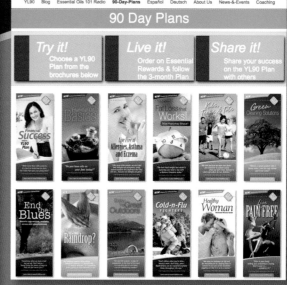
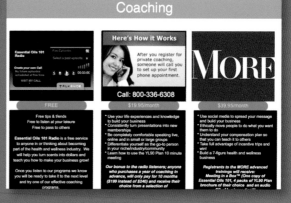